ALTERNATIVE
REMEDIES
FOR COMMON
AILMENTS

TIME
LIFE
BOOKS

ALEXANDRIA, VIRGINIA

TIME® LIFE BOOKS

TIME-LIFE BOOKS IS A DIVISION OF TIME LIFE INC.

TIME LIFE INC.
PRESIDENT and CEO: George Artandi

TIME-LIFE CUSTOM PUBLISHING
Vice President and Publisher: Terry Newell
Vice President of Sales and Marketing: Neil Levin
Director of Special Sales: Liz Ziehl
Editor for Special Markets: Anna Burgard
Production Manager: Carolyn Bounds
Quality Assurance Manager: James King
Special Contributors: Ruth Thompson, Thunder Hill Graphics
(production), Celia Beattie (proofreading), Judy Davis (index)

This book is an adaptation of the Time-Life edition
The Alternative Advisor ©1997

Director of Editorial Development: Jennifer Pearce
Editor: Robert Somerville
Deputy Editor: Tina S. McDowell
Design Director: Tina Taylor
Text Editor: Jim Watson
Associate Editors/Research and Writing: Nancy Blodgett, Stephanie
Summers Henke
Technical Art Assistant: Dana R. Magsumbol
Senior Copyeditors: Anne Farr, Mary Beth Oelkers-Keegan
Picture Coordinator: Lisa Groseclose
Editorial Assistant: Patricia D. Whiteford

Library of Congress Cataloging-in-Publication Data
Time-Life alternative remedies for common ailments.
p. cm.
Includes index.
ISBN 0-7370-1105-X
1. Alternative medicine—Popular works.
2. Self-care, Health.
I. Time-Life Books.
R733.T56 1998
615.5—dc21   98-2853 CIP

Books produced by Time-Life Custom Publishing are available at
special bulk discount for promotional and premium use. Custom
adaptations can also be created to meet your specific marketing
goals. Call 1-800-323-5255.

The textual and visual decriptions of medical conditions and treatment options in this book should be considered as a reference source only; they are not intended to substitute for a healthcare practitioner's diagnosis, advice, and treatment. Always consult your physician or a qualified practitioner for proper medical care.

Before using any drug or natural medicine mentioned in this book, be sure to check with your healthcare practitioner, and check the product packaging or other reliable source of information for any warnings or cautions. You should keep in mind that herbal remedies are not as strictly regulated as drugs.

Cover photographs courtesy of PhotoDisc
Cover design by Anna Burgard

Table of Contents

$\mathcal{O}$ntroduction

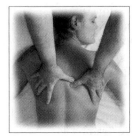 Alternative therapies are used with varying degrees of success to treat virtually every known medical condition. Depending on the type and severity of the disorder, the benefits range from complete cures to relief of symptoms such as pain, dizziness, and nausea. In many cases, alternative remedies are used alone or in combination with other techniques to complement or boost the effectiveness of conventional treatments. It is important to note, however, that while many ailments can be treated effectively with alternative therapies, some disorders require the care of a conventional medical doctor. Listed here are more than 40 ailments—some of them minor and merely annoying, others chronic and potentially life threatening—for which various forms of alternative medicine have proved to be beneficial in one way or another.

For the most part, the ailments in this book are listed individually by name in alphabetical order. In a few cases, however, similar or related disorders have been grouped under a single heading. "Athletic Injuries," for example, contains information about a number of common sports-related complaints, from ligament sprains and muscle strains to bone fractures and joint dislocations. Various skin disorders, including psoriasis, dermatitis, and skin cancer, are discussed in "Rashes and Skin Problems." Conditions that cause persistent discomfort in the back, joints, neck, and other areas of the body are covered in the entry labeled "Pain, Chronic." If you have trouble locating an ailment entry, you should be able to find it easily in the index.

Each entry begins with a general overview of the ailment, briefly touching on such aspects as its cause or causes, how it affects the body, and the prospects for recovery. Following the introduction is a section entitled Treatment Options, which is a detailed list of alternative therapies that may be useful in caring for the condition; information on conventional medical care is included as necessary. Here you'll find specific information and suggestions that will help you decide which alternative avenue to pursue. Techniques discussed under the heading Home Remedies are simple but effective ways you can treat the ailment yourself using materials you have around the house or can easily obtain. The section headed Prevention suggests steps you can take to lessen your chances of a recurrence of the condition or of developing it in the first place.

A permanent fixture at the beginning of each entry is the Symptoms box, a summary of the ailment's characteristic warning signs. Immediately below it is the Call Your Doctor If box, which describes symptoms that are serious enough to warrant the attention of a physician or, in some cases, a trip to the emergency room. Important warnings about the disease or its treatment appear in a Caution box, located in the bottom left corner of the opening page. Other boxes placed throughout the entry shed additional light on the ailment, separating fact from myth, explaining important new findings, or pointing out other matters of interest. Many entries also feature drawings that show affected areas of the body (sometimes revealing the ailment's damage-causing mechanism), or that give step-by-step instructions on how to perform certain therapeutic techniques, such as acupressure or yoga.

As it turns out, not every alternative therapy is appropriate for every individual. You'll find that some work better for you than others; or you may discover that a combination of techniques—say, herbal therapy and yoga—produces the most effective results. The best way to learn which approach is best suited to you and your condition is to consult your healthcare practitioner. And never hesitate to consult a physician if circumstances warrant. ■

$\mathscr{A}$llergies

Symptoms

- Sneezing, wheezing, nasal congestion, and coughing indicate asthma, or drug or respiratory allergies.

- Itchy eyes, mouth, and throat are symptoms of respiratory allergies.

- Stomachache, frequent indigestion, and heartburn are signs of food sensitivities.

- Irritated, itchy, reddening, or swelling skin is associated with drug, food, and insect-sting allergies.

- Stiffness, pain, and swelling of joints may indicate food or drug allergies.

- Fatigue or feeling run-down, difficulty concentrating, emotional upset or irritability, or difficulty sleeping may be associated with food allergies or seasonal allergies such as hay fever.

Call Your Doctor If

- you have violent stomach cramps, vomiting, bloating, or diarrhea; this could point to a serious food or other allergic reaction or food poisoning.

- breathing becomes extremely difficult or painful; you may be experiencing an asthma episode, another serious allergic reaction, or a heart attack. Get emergency medical treatment.

- you suddenly develop skin welts accompanied by intense flushing and itching; your heart may also be beating rapidly. These symptoms may indicate the onset of anaphylactic shock, an extremely serious allergic reaction *(box, opposite)*. Get emergency medical treatment.

T*he term "allergy" applies to an abnormal reaction by your immune system to a substance that is usually safe. Allergies come in many forms and range from mildly bothersome to life threatening.*

The immune system protects the body from foreign substances—known as antigens—by producing antibodies and other chemicals to fight them. Usually, the immune system ignores benign substances, such as food, and fights only dangerous ones, such as bacteria. A person develops an allergic reaction when the immune system cannot tell the good from the bad and releases a type of chemical called histamine to attack the harmless substance as if it were a threat. Histamine produces many of the symptoms associated with allergies. Allergens, or substances that may trigger allergic reactions, range from pollen to pet dander to penicillin.

Most allergic reactions are not serious, but some, such as anaphylaxis, can be fatal (see box, below, right). Only a few allergies can be cured outright, but the symptoms can be relieved. If your allergy is severe, it is vital that you visit a conventional medical doctor and get immediate treatment on an emergency basis.

Treatment Options

Since allergies can be hard to diagnose and are in many cases incurable, alternative remedies for them have become quite popular. But for severe allergies, or for emergencies, you must see a conventional physician. Blood tests can detect food allergies.

Aromatherapy

To relieve nasal congestion, try mixing 1 drop each of the oils of lavender *(Lavandula angustifolia)* and niaouli *(Melaleuca viridiflora)*, and 1 tsp of a carrier oil such as sweet almond or sunflower; massage into the skin around your sinuses once a day. Eucalyptus globulus *(E. globulus)* and peppermint *(Mentha piperita)* oils also act as decongestants; dab on a handkerchief and inhale.

Chinese Medicine

Chinese herbalists use the mixture *Bi Yan Pian* for allergies with a runny nose, as well as a commercially prepared mixture of herbs, found in many natural food stores, called Hayfever. Acupuncture, too, may be helpful; consult a qualified practitioner.

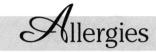 Allergies

Herbal Therapies

Infusions of chamomile *(Matricaria recutita)*, elder *(Sambucus nigra)* flower, eyebright *(Euphrasia officinalis)*, garlic *(Allium sativum)*, goldenrod *(Solidago virgaurea)*, nettle *(Urtica dioica)*, and yarrow *(Achillea millefolium)* have antimucus and anti-inflammatory effects. Some herbs, such as nettles, may cause an allergic reaction; use with caution.

Ginger tea can help reduce sinus inflammation. Simmer 2 tsp chopped or grated ginger *(Zingiber officinale)* in 2 cups water for 20 minutes. Breathe in the steam for five to seven minutes; repeat several times each day, until your symptoms subside.

Homeopathy

For a runny nose, itchy throat, and sneezing, a practitioner might suggest *Arsenicum album* (12c) or *Sabadilla* (30c); for chronic thick mucus, *Pulsatilla* (12c); for a runny nose, sore upper lip, and itchy eyes, *Allium cepa* (12c); for hives, allergic swelling—including painful joints, or allergic reactions to bee stings—*Apis* (12c); for indigestion with stuffiness and runny nose, *Nux vomica* (30c).

Nutrition and Diet

Vitamin C and bioflavonoids (found in the white pith of citrus fruits) act as natural antihistamines, so you should increase your citrus intake or take 1,000 mg of vitamin C three times daily. Vitamins A

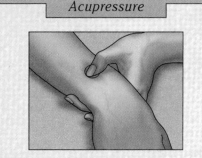

Acupressure

Triple Warmer 5 • *Use this point to help fortify the immune system. Center your thumb on the top of your forearm, two thumb widths from the wrist joint, and press firmly. Repeat on the other arm.*

and B complex appear to stimulate the immune system. Products made with bee pollen and royal jelly may alleviate or eliminate respiratory symptoms but should not be taken if you are allergic to bee stings. For food allergies, read labels carefully and make sure you know what foods to avoid.

Avoid all stimulants, such as caffeinated beverages and white sugar, and decaffeinated drinks; these substances can overstimulate the immune system, making allergies worse.

Prevention

Respiratory allergies: Install a high-efficiency air cleaner to help remove pollen and mold spores, and use an air conditioner in your home and car during warm seasons to keep pollen out; regularly clean damp areas with bleach to kill molds. Consider hiring a special cleaning service to rid furniture and upholstery of dust mites. Isolate (or, if you can stand it, get rid of) your pets and keep them outside as much as possible. Regular baths for your pet will help reduce dander.

Food allergies: Avoid foods that are highly allergenic, such as dairy products, wheat, corn, soybean, and citrus fruits. Instead of dairy products, try tofu-based foods. Always check food labels for additives that are known allergens, such as yellow food dye no. 5 and gum arabic. ■

OF SPECIAL INTEREST

What Triggers Anaphylactic Shock?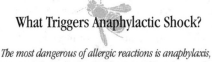

The most dangerous of allergic reactions is anaphylaxis, or anaphylactic shock, which begins within minutes after exposure and advances quickly. Although any allergen can trigger anaphylactic shock, the most common are insect stings, foods such as shellfish and nuts, and injections of certain drugs. Standard emergency treatment includes an injection of epinephrine to open airways and blood vessels; in severe cases, cardiopulmonary resuscitation (CPR) may be needed.

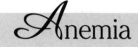Anemia

Symptoms

- Weakness, fatigue, and a general feeling of malaise; you may be mildly anemic.

- Your lips look bluish, your skin is pasty or yellowish, and your gums, nail beds, eyelid linings, or palm creases are pale; you are almost certainly anemic.

- In addition to feeling weak and tired, you are frequently out of breath, faint, or dizzy; you may have severe anemia.

- Your tongue burns; you may have vitamin B_{12} anemia.

- Your tongue feels unusually slick and you experience movement or balance problems, tingling in the extremities, confusion, depression, or memory loss; you may have pernicious anemia.

- Other possible symptoms: headache, insomnia, decreased appetite, poor concentration, and an irregular heartbeat.

Call Your Doctor If

- you have the symptoms of pernicious anemia; this disorder can damage the spinal cord.

- you have been taking iron supplements and experience symptoms such as vomiting, bloody diarrhea, fever, jaundice, lethargy, or seizures; you may be suffering from iron overload, which can be life threatening, especially in children.

Anemia, in which body tissues are deprived of oxygen, is caused by a reduction in the number of circulating red blood cells or by inadequate amounts of the essential protein hemoglobin. The severity can range from mild to life threatening. Anemia can occur if large amounts of blood are lost or if something interferes with the production of red blood cells or accelerates their destruction. Because hemoglobin is the main component of red blood cells and the carrier for oxygen molecules, anemia also occurs if the hemoglobin supply is insufficient or if the hemoglobin itself is dysfunctional.

More than 400 forms of anemia have been identified. The disorder may arise from a number of underlying conditions, some of which may be hereditary, but in many cases poor diet is to blame. Iron deficiency anemia, the leading form, occurs when the body does not store enough iron, the chief raw material of hemoglobin. The only way to know what kind of anemia you have is to ask your doctor to run tests on a sample of your blood.

Treatment Options

Some remedies treat anemia by promoting better circulation, others by increasing iron absorption, stimulating digestion, or adjusting the diet to include more iron- or vitamin-rich foods.

Herbal Therapies

In the history of folk medicine, bitter substances have always been thought to stimulate digestion and thereby promote the absorption of valuable nutrients. The bitter herb gentian *(Gentiana lutea)* is a popular remedy in Europe for a number of nutritionally based ailments, including anemia. Gentian can be brewed into a tea or ingested in the form of a commercially available alcoholic extract. Dandelion *(Taraxacum officinale)* is also thought to benefit people with anemia, simply because it is rich in vitamins and minerals. Other iron-rich herbs include parsley *(Petroselinum crispum)* and nettle *(Urtica dioica)*.

In traditional Chinese medicine, anemia is a condition known as deficient blood. Treatment might involve acupuncture and herbal therapies. Research suggests that Asian ginseng *(Panax ginseng)* is useful as a general tonic to counteract

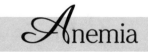

Anemia

anemia-induced fatigue. Dong quai *(Angelica sinensis)*, another Asian herb used medicinally for thousands of years, is a blood tonic. For anemic patients who have a gray cast, a Chinese herbalist might recommend a combination of dong quai and Chinese foxglove root *(Rehmannia glutinosa)*. For patients with a stark white complexion, the remedy might be a mixture of ginseng and astragalus *(Astragalus membranaceus)*. After diagnosing a person with anemia, a Chinese medicine practitioner might recommend the following herbal formulas: *Ba Zhen Wan* (Eight Treasure Pills) or *Shi Quan Da Bu Wan* (Ten Complete Great Tonifying Pills).

■ Homeopathy
Consult a professional homeopath for an evaluation that will determine which substances are most suitable for treating your type of anemia.

■ Nutrition and Diet
Adjusting your diet is the easiest, most healthful, and longest-lasting way to combat any anemia linked to nutritional deficiency. A vast array of foods can boost your iron count, including enriched breads and cereals, rice, potatoes, carrots, broccoli, tomatoes, dried beans, blackstrap molasses, lean red meat, liver, poultry, dried fruits, almonds, and shellfish. Research indicates that iron from animal sources is absorbed more readily than plant iron. Evidence also suggests that vitamin C and copper help the body absorb iron.

If you're low on folic acid, a key player in red blood cell production, step up your consumption of citrus fruits, mushrooms, dark green vegetables, liver, eggs, milk, and bulking agents like wheat germ and brewer's yeast. Also, pumpkin is an excellent source of folate, which is the vitamin B complex component of folic acid. Keep in mind that folic acid is destroyed by heat and light, so fruits and vegetables should be eaten fresh and cooked as little as possible.

Vegetarians are at risk for vitamin B_{12} anemia because this vitamin is found only in animal products and in some fermented foods. If you are a vegetarian, you need to include in your diet dairy products and eggs or fermented foods such as miso and tofu, or take a daily supplement of B_{12}.

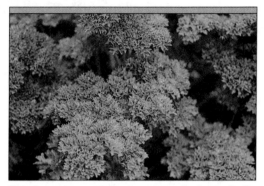

Parsley • *A versatile and nutritious herb, parsley is a good natural source of iron and thus can be useful in treating iron deficiency anemia. Parsley is also rich in vitamin C, which promotes iron absorption in the body.*

Home Remedies

■ Keep track of the foods you eat and find out whether they are rich in iron, folic acid, or vitamin B_{12}. You might be surprised to learn that some of the foods you eat are preventing the absorption of needed nutrients.

■ Don't drink caffeinated or decaffeinated tea, coffee, or cola with meals; caffeine inhibits iron absorption, as does the tannin in black tea. The acids in decaffeinated beverages can also be a problem. You should, however, drink citrus juices, because they are rich in vitamin C, which promotes iron absorption.

■ Consider taking a daily multivitamin. Be sure to consult a doctor or nutritionist before taking iron supplements; excess amounts of iron in your system can be harmful.

Prevention

■ Avoid excessive consumption of alcohol. Chronic drinking can undermine proper nutrition and interfere with the digestive system's ability to absorb folic acid, necessary for the production of red blood cells.

■ Take a daily multivitamin to maintain a healthful balance of vitamins and minerals. ■

Arthritis

Symptoms

■ Pain and progressive stiffness without noticeable swelling, chills, or fever during normal activities probably indicate the gradual onset of osteoarthritis.

■ Painful swelling, inflammation, and stiffness in the arms, legs, wrists, or fingers in the same joints on both sides of the body, especially on awakening, may be signs of rheumatoid arthritis.

■ Fever, joint inflammation, tenderness, and sharp pain, sometimes accompanied by chills and associated with an injury or another illness, may indicate infectious arthritis.

■ In children, intermittent fever, loss of appetite, weight loss, anemia, or blotchy rash on the arms and legs may signal juvenile rheumatoid arthritis.

Call Your Doctor If

■ the pain and stiffness come on quickly, whether from an injury or an unknown cause; you may be experiencing the onset of rheumatoid arthritis.

■ the pain is accompanied by fever; you may have infectious arthritis.

■ you notice pain and stiffness in your arms, legs, or back after sitting for short periods or after a night's sleep; you may be developing osteoarthritis or another arthritic condition.

■ a child develops pain or a rash on armpits, knees, wrists, and ankles, or has fever swings, poor appetite, and weight loss; the child may have juvenile rheumatoid arthritis.

A lthough the term is applied to a wide variety of disorders, arthritis strictly means the inflammation of a joint, whether as the result of a disease, an infection, a genetic defect, or some other cause.

Major Types of Arthritis

Rheumatoid arthritis, also called rheumatism or synovitis, tends to affect people over the age of 40 and women two to three times as frequently as men. It is characterized by inflammation and pain in the hands—especially the knuckles and second joints—as well as in the arms, legs, and feet, and by general fatigue and sleeplessness. It can also cause systemic damage to other parts of the body, including the heart, lungs, eyes, nerves, and muscles. Rheumatoid arthritis in older people may eventually cause the hands and feet to become gnarled and misshapen as muscles weaken, tendons shrink, and the ends of bones become abnormally enlarged.

Juvenile rheumatoid arthritis, or Still's disease, is characterized by chronic fever and anemia. It can also affect the heart, lungs, eyes, and nervous system. Arthritic episodes in children younger than five can last for several weeks and may recur, although the symptoms tend to be less severe in recurrent attacks. Most affected children recover from the disease fully with no ill effects.

Infectious arthritis refers to various ailments that affect larger arm and leg joints as well as the fingers or toes. Arthritic infection is usually a complication of an injury or of another disease and is much less common than arthritic conditions that come on with age.

Osteoarthritis, or degenerative joint disease, refers to the pain and inflammation that can result from the systematic loss of bone tissue in the joints. It is the most common form of arthritis, particularly in the elderly. In osteoarthritis, the protective cartilage at the ends of bones in joints—especially in the spine and legs—gradually wears away. The inner bone surfaces become exposed and rub together. In some cases, bony spurs develop on the edges of joints, causing damage to muscles and nerves, pain, deformity, and difficulty in movement.

Although the mechanism of osteoarthritis is unknown, some people appear to have a genetic

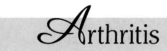 Arthritis

predisposition to degenerative bone disorders. In rare cases, congenital bone deformation appears at an early age. Misuse of anabolic steroids, which are popular among some athletes, can also bring on early osteoarthritic degeneration.

In many people the onset of osteoarthritis is gradual and is not seriously debilitating, although it can change the shape and size of bones. In other people, bony growths and gnarled joints may cause painful muscle inflammation or nerve damage, along with changes in posture and mobility.

Treatment Options

Sometimes arthritic damage can be slowed or stopped, but in most cases the damage continues as the disease runs its course, regardless of the use of drugs or other therapies. Because medical science has not found any full cures for the various kinds of arthritis, many people turn to alternative treatments to ease their pain and disability. While the effectiveness of few alternative approaches can be substantiated, research indicates that some of these methods, such as meditation, self-hypnosis, guided imagery, and relaxation techniques, can play a significant role in treating arthritic ailments.

■ **Acupressure and Acupuncture**
Some arthritis patients find that these therapies, administered by a trained practitioner, offer effective relief from the pain of rheumatoid arthritis or osteoarthritis for several weeks or months.

Joint Degeneration

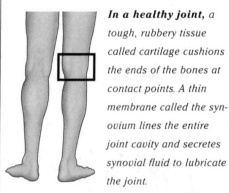

In a healthy joint, a tough, rubbery tissue called cartilage cushions the ends of the bones at contact points. A thin membrane called the synovium lines the entire joint cavity and secretes synovial fluid to lubricate the joint.

In rheumatoid arthritis, the synovial membrane becomes thickened and inflamed. The inflammation causes cartilage to break down at the pivot point of the joint, while excess synovial fluid causes the cavity to swell.

Osteoarthritis—also called wear-and-tear arthritis—results from gradual deterioration of cartilage in the joint after years of use. Without the protective cartilage, the bones begin to rub together, creating friction and pain.

BONE
CARTILAGE
SYNOVIAL FLUID
SYNOVIAL MEMBRANE

SYNOVIAL MEMBRANE

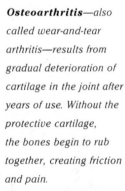

INFLAMED MEMBRANE

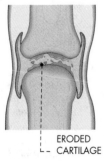

ERODED CARTILAGE

11

CONTINUED

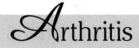

Arthritis

■ Body Work

Soft-tissue massage around affected joints or com-passionate touching can have a comforting effect on those who suffer from arthritis. Manipulation by a therapist constitutes passive exercise for people unable to perform vigorous exercise. Besides mak-ing a patient feel better physically, sympathetically administered touch therapy can help soothe the emotional effects of chronic illness. Further, stud-ies suggest that relieving stress and tension has a positive influence on the body's hormonal balance.

■ Chiropractic

A chiropractor may manipulate the spine and other arthritic joints very carefully to relieve pain and help reestablish normal use. A program for arthri-tis may also include exercise, physiotherapy, and nutritional interventions.

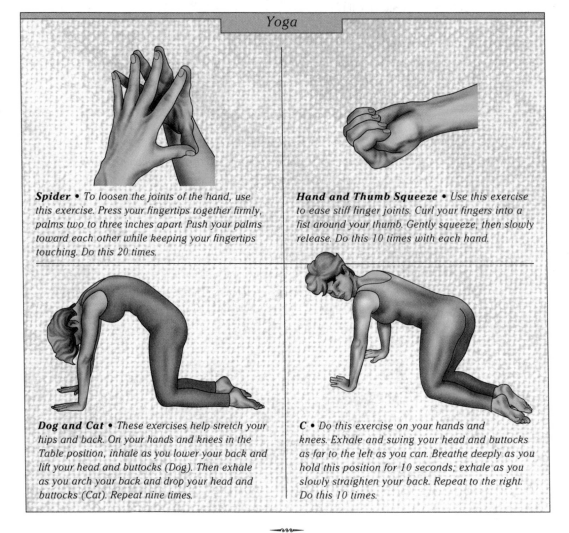

Yoga

Spider • *To loosen the joints of the hand, use this exercise. Press your fingertips together firmly, palms two to three inches apart. Push your palms toward each other while keeping your fingertips touching. Do this 20 times.*

Hand and Thumb Squeeze • *Use this exercise to ease stiff finger joints. Curl your fingers into a fist around your thumb. Gently squeeze, then slowly release. Do this 10 times with each hand.*

Dog and Cat • *These exercises help stretch your hips and back. On your hands and knees in the Table position, inhale as you lower your back and lift your head and buttocks (Dog). Then exhale as you arch your back and drop your head and buttocks (Cat). Repeat nine times.*

C • *Do this exercise on your hands and knees. Exhale and swing your head and buttocks as far to the left as you can. Breathe deeply as you hold this position for 10 seconds; exhale as you slowly straighten your back. Repeat to the right. Do this 10 times.*

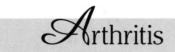

Arthritis

Flower Remedy

To help relieve inflammation, apply Rescue Remedy cream, a Bach flower remedy, to the inflamed or painful area three or four times a day.

Herbal Therapies

Among the various remedies herbalists recommend to relieve pain is a 5-ml tincture made from 2 parts willow (*Salix* spp.) bark and 1 part each of black cohosh *(Cimicifuga racemosa)* and nettle *(Urtica dioica),* taken three times a day. To relieve muscle tension, rub a tincture of lobelia *(Lobelia inflata)* and cramp bark *(Viburnum opulus)* on the affected area. The Chinese herbal formula *Du Huo Ji Sheng Wan* is useful for some types of arthritis.

Homeopathy

For chronic osteoarthritis and rheumatoid arthritis, constitutional remedies may be prescribed after consultation with a trained homeopathic practitioner. Homeopathic remedies to relieve immediate pain and joint stiffness may include *Rhus toxicodendron* or *Bryonia.*

Hydrotherapy

Swimming or other water exercise, preferably in a heated pool, can improve joint movement and muscle strength; the water helps support the body and reduce the stress of gravity.

Massage

Massage can soothe pain, relax stiff muscles, and reduce the swelling that accompanies arthritis. Massage and gentle stretching help maintain a joint's range of motion.

Nutrition and Diet

Avoiding specific foods can stop arthritic symptoms associated with allergies, especially allergies to grains, nuts, meats, eggs, and dairy products. Use trial and error, preferably under the supervision of an allergist.

Avoid caffeinated and decaffeinated beverages and sugary foods, which tighten the tendons and cause blood vessels to constrict; this increases pain and decreases flexibility.

Some practitioners recommend cutting out plants in the nightshade family: tomato, potato, eggplant, and pepper. They believe the alkaloids in these foods inhibit formation of the collagen that makes up cartilage. Be patient—it may take up to six months before you see an improvement. Once you determine that these foods do affect you, eat them only occasionally. If your symptoms don't improve after six months, then nightshades aren't a factor in your arthritis.

Low-fat, low-protein vegetarian diets may ease the discomfort of rheumatoid arthritis. Good results are reported from eliminating partially hydrogenated fats and polyunsaturated vegetable oils and supplementing the diet with flax oil, sardines, and other oily fish as a source of omega-3 fatty acids.

Vitamin therapy may relieve certain arthritic symptoms. Beta carotene (vitamin A) has an antioxidant effect on cells, neutralizing destructive molecules called free radicals. Vitamins C, B_6, and E, as well as zinc, are thought to enhance collagen production and the repair of connective tissue. Vitamin C may also be advised for people taking aspirin, which depletes the body's vitamin C balance. Niacin (vitamin B_3) may also be helpful, although excessive use may aggravate liver problems. Always take vitamin supplements under professional guidance, since overdoses of some vitamin compounds can have side effects or undesirable interactions with drugs.

Some therapists recommend cherries or dark red berries to stimulate the production of collagen, essential to cartilage repair. The nutritional supplement glucosamine sulfate may also help.

Home Remedies

Heat and rest—traditional remedies for arthritic pain—are very effective in the short term for most people. Weight control is important, especially when arthritis strikes the lower back and legs.

If arthritic pain comes on unexpectedly, supplement an over-the-counter painkiller with dry heat from a heating pad or moist heat in the form of a hot bath or a hot-water bottle wrapped in a towel. However, do not use heat if you have infectious arthritis. For all types of arthritis, regular exercise is important to keep the joints mobile. ■

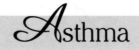Asthma

Symptoms

- Restlessness or insomnia.

- Increasing, but relatively painless, tightness in chest.

- Mild to moderate shortness of breath.

- When breathing, a wheezing or whistling sound that can range from faint to clearly audible.

- Coughing, sometimes accompanied by phlegm.

Call Your Doctor If

- you or another person is experiencing an episode of asthma for the first time; asthma is a chronic condition and can be quite serious if not treated properly.

- the prescribed asthma medicine does not work in the time it is supposed to; you need a new prescription, or you may be suffering from a severe episode.

- you or the person with asthma has a suffocating feeling, making it difficult to talk; nostrils flare, the skin between the ribs appears sucked in, and the lips or the skin under the nails looks grayish or bluish. These are all signs of extreme oxygen deprivation. Get immediate emergency treatment.

Yoga

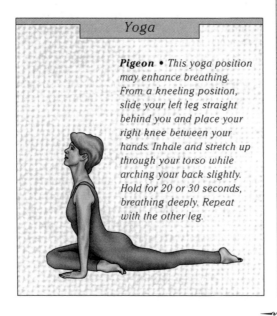

Pigeon • This yoga position may enhance breathing. From a kneeling position, slide your left leg straight behind you and place your right knee between your hands. Inhale and stretch up through your torso while arching your back slightly. Hold for 20 or 30 seconds, breathing deeply. Repeat with the other leg.

A sthma is a chronic respiratory disease that, like bronchitis and emphysema, causes a tightening of the chest and difficulty in breathing. In the case of asthma, however, these symptoms are not always present. They come in episodes set off by various environmental or emotional triggers, such as pollen, animal dander, tobacco smoke, and stress. Episodes can be brought on by a variety of factors working alone or in combination. Allergies are the primary offenders. Some people with asthma experience only mild and infrequent attacks; for them the condition is an occasional inconvenience. For others, episodes can be frequent and serious, requiring emergency medical treatment. If you have asthma, you should seek the help of a doctor before trying alternative therapies.

Treatment Options

Many people have reported success with alternative asthma treatments, but even advocates recommend these methods only as complements to conventional therapies. Once diagnosed, asthma should be monitored by a physician; serious episodes require conventional medical attention.

Acupuncture

Medical studies suggest that acupuncture may help alleviate asthma symptoms. The procedure should be carried out only by a licensed acupuncturist.

Aromatherapy

Essential oils such as eucalyptus globulus (*E. globulus*), aniseed (*Pimpinella anisum*), lavender (*Lavandula angustifolia*), pine (*Pinus sylvestris*), and rosemary (*Rosmarinus officinalis*) may help ease breathing and relieve nasal congestion. Inhaled through the nose, a few drops of one of the oils or a mixture of several dabbed on a handkerchief or tissue can help ease breathing during a mild episode of asthma. If you feel congested at other times (not during an episode), mix a few drops of essential oil in a sink full of hot water, cover your head with a towel, and inhale the fragrant steam through your nose. Use caution with essential oils if you have not used them before; in some circumstances they can precipitate an attack. Try applying them topically first before inhaling.

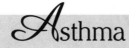
Asthma

Herbal Therapies

Elecampane *(Inula helenium)*, a root that acts as a soothing expectorant, may help clear the body of excess mucus. To prepare an infusion, shred the root to yield 1 tsp and add a full cup of cold water; let the infusion stand for 10 hours, then strain and drink it hot three times daily. An infusion made from mullein *(Verbascum thapsus)* is recommended for soothing the mucous membranes, especially during nighttime episodes.

One formula recommended by practitioners of Chinese medicine is cinnamon twig decoction. Mix 9 grams cinnamon *(Cinnamomum cassia)* twigs, 9 grams white peony root, 9 grams ginger *(Zingiber officinale)*, 6 grams Chinese licorice *(Glycyrrhiza uralensis)*, and 12 pieces Chinese dates; steep the mixture in cold water, then bring to a boil. Drink it hot.

Homeopathy

A number of homeopathic remedies are available for treating asthma symptoms. Following are just a few: To help calm restlessness and anxiety, take *Arsenicum album* (30c) as required. For symptoms that worsen at night or during cold weather, or that come on very suddenly, take *Aconite* (6c) as required. For symptoms exacerbated by dampness, take *Natrum sulphuricum* (6c) as required. For more remedies, consult a licensed homeopathic or naturopathic physician.

Reflexology

Working the reflexology areas corresponding to the lungs, chest, diaphragm, and adrenals may help relieve an attack.

Yoga

Yoga can help you learn to breathe deeply and to relax, thereby helping you deal more effectively with stress, a common trigger for asthma.

Prevention

- Learn to identify your triggers: Keep a diary detailing all the environmental and emotional factors that affect you every day over the course of several months. When you have an asthma attack, go back to your diary to see

Asthmatic Airways

Air travels down the trachea and into the lungs through branching tubes called bronchioles, which normally are lined with a thin mucous membrane. For people with asthma, certain conditions or inhaled substances can act as triggers, prompting the release of chemicals that cause the bronchioles to constrict and produce excess mucus. The clogged airways trap air and make breathing difficult.

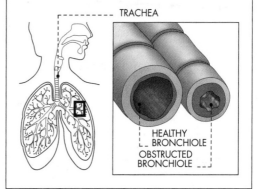

TRACHEA

HEALTHY BRONCHIOLE
OBSTRUCTED BRONCHIOLE

which factor, or combination of factors, might have contributed to it.

- Avoid foods and drinks that have high concentrations of sulfites, such as beer, wine, wine vinegar, instant tea, grape juice, lemon juice, grapes, fresh shrimp, pizza dough, dried fruits (such as apricots and apples), canned vegetables, instant potatoes, corn syrup, fruit topping, molasses, and foods found in salad bars. Some nutritionists recommend that you also steer clear of foods that cause excess mucus production, such as milk.

- A daily dose of B-complex vitamins (50 to 100 mg) and magnesium (400 to 600 mg) may help reduce the frequency and severity of asthma episodes. ■

A

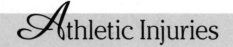

Athletic Injuries

Symptoms

- Pain, discomfort, restricted movement, tenderness, and possible swelling may be indicative of some form of muscle or ligament injury, such as a sprain or strain.

- Pain, swelling, tenderness, and deformity may indicate a fracture.

- Pain, restricted movement, misshapen appearance, and swelling in a joint are symptoms of a dislocation.

- Localized pain just below the kneecap may be a sign of patellar tendinitis. In adolescents, the condition may indicate Osgood-Schlatter disease if accompanied by swelling.

- Pain in the elbow, often accompanied by tenderness in the inner or outer portion of the elbow and forearm, and possibly a weak and painful grasp, may be an indication of epicondylitis.

Call Your Doctor If

- your muscles gradually become weak for no apparent reason; you may have a neurological problem or another disorder of immediate concern.

- you experience chronic muscle cramps. Although most often benign, this may be a sign of serious problems such as blood clotting, restricted blood flow, or nerve damage.

- you think your swelling or puffiness is caused by a fracture, dislocation, ligament or muscle tear, or cartilage damage. If not treated by a physician in a timely manner, the affected area could suffer permanent damage.

 very family has seen its share of injuries tracing to athletic endeavors or, ironically, the pursuit of physical fitness. For the most part, athletic injuries are a result of stress put on bones or muscles. Most common are injuries to soft tissue—muscles, tendons, and ligaments.

A dislocation occurs when two bones are jolted apart at a joint and is often accompanied by a ligament tear in the joint. The pain is caused by the severe stretching of soft tissues.

A fracture is either simple (closed)—in which the broken bone remains beneath the skin surface and does minimal damage to surrounding tissues—or compound (open), in which the bone protrudes through the skin. The ankle, hand, wrist, and collarbone are common sites of fracture.

INJURIES TO THE UPPER BODY

Shoulder injuries are common in sports that require throwing motions or intense contact. Dislocations are most common in the shoulder joint. Acromioclavicular joint (AC) separation occurs when the ligaments that support the collarbone are torn as a result of sudden impact on the side of the shoulder or on an outstretched arm. The rotator cuff is where four muscles meet and attach to the humerus; overuse of the shoulder, perhaps as a result of sports that require overhead motion like that in a tennis serve, may inflame or tear tendons in the area, causing rotator cuff tendinitis.

Epicondylitis affects the elbow and typically occurs in sports requiring frequent wrist manipulation and forearm rotation. The lateral (affecting the outer elbow) form is tennis elbow. Medial epicondylitis, caused by repetitive arm motion, as in pitching a baseball, involves the inner elbow.

The sudden tearing of muscle fibers that may occur after excessive athletic activity and the consequent accumulation of fluid in the muscle that causes pain, tenderness, and local swelling characterize a charley horse.

INJURIES TO THE LOWER BODY

Lower back injuries, such as muscle tears, are common in sports that involve a lot of bending. The

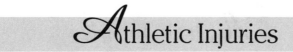thletic Injuries

high velocity and full-contact nature of hockey and football frequently cause neck and spine injuries, such as a herniated disk, in which an intervertebral disk protrudes from the spinal column.

Intense leg movement, including twisting and spreading, may tear the adductor muscle, causing groin strain. This muscle connects the leg with the pubic bone.

The knees are involved in some of the most common lower body injuries. Continual jumping may result in tearing of the tendon just below the kneecap (patella), causing patellar tendinitis, or jumper's knee. The knees may also suffer from other injuries, such as tears of the meniscus, a piece of cartilage in the knee joint between the femur and tibia.

Increased interest in jogging and cross training has resulted in a parallel rise in leg injuries, including shin splints, tendinitis, and stress fractures, especially in the tibia or fibula bones. If continually exposed to stress from prolonged standing, running, or walking, a stress fracture may result in a larger fracture.

The foot often falls victim to injury because it must support the weight of the entire body. Plantar fasciitis often affects inexperienced runners, causing pain along the inner heel and along the arch of

---

OF SPECIAL INTEREST

Growing Pains

Osgood-Schlatter disease is a condition associated with sudden growth spurts in adolescence (usually in boys ages 10 to 14). It is characterized by pain and swelling below the kneecap, where the patellar tendon attaches to the shinbone. The quadriceps muscle, located at the front of the thigh, continually pulls on the affected tendon, causing the disorder. Osgood-Schlatter disease persists for six months to a year and usually clears up completely without treatment. However, as long as your child suffers from symptoms, activities such as running, jumping, and squatting should be kept to a minimum, if not eliminated completely.

Common Sports Injuries

The highlighted areas below show some of the sites of common injuries sustained from sports or other physical activity. The best way to prevent an athletic injury is to be in good physical condition and to stretch for several minutes before and after exercising. Never attempt to "play through" pain—doing so may cause more-extensive injury and lengthen the time needed for complete healing.

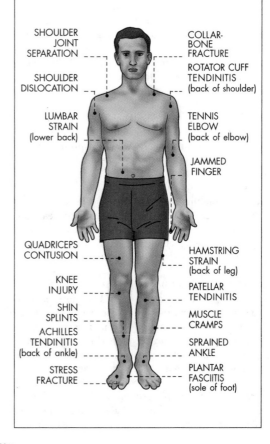

SHOULDER JOINT SEPARATION

SHOULDER DISLOCATION

LUMBAR STRAIN (lower back)

QUADRICEPS CONTUSION

KNEE INJURY

SHIN SPLINTS

ACHILLES TENDINITIS (back of ankle)

STRESS FRACTURE

COLLARBONE FRACTURE

ROTATOR CUFF TENDINITIS (back of shoulder)

TENNIS ELBOW (back of elbow)

JAMMED FINGER

HAMSTRING STRAIN (back of leg)

PATELLAR TENDINITIS

MUSCLE CRAMPS

SPRAINED ANKLE

PLANTAR FASCIITIS (sole of foot)

CONTINUED

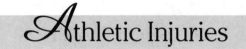

Athletic Injuries

the foot, sometimes accompanied by stiffness and numbness in the heel. A similar problem, march fracture, develops in the bones of the foot when extreme stress (as in running) is continually placed on the ball of the foot.

Treatment Options

Most minor soft-tissue injuries are best treated with RICE: rest, ice, compression, and elevation. The following alternative therapies can help alleviate the pain and other symptoms of an athletic injury, but severe injuries require a doctor's care.

Acupuncture
Administered by a professional, acupuncture may be helpful in treating athletic injuries and soothing the body after strenuous training. It has been shown to reduce pain and swelling, and it may also speed recovery of injured muscles, tendons, and ligaments. For best results, acupuncture should be performed as soon as possible after injury occurs.

Body Work
Administered by a professional, the Alexander technique, Rolfing, and the Feldenkrais method may be useful, particularly when the problem involves body structure or movement patterns.

Chinese Medicine
Various combinations of Chinese herbs, tailored to the individual's condition, can be used to treat athletic injuries. Herbal liniments often recommended by practitioners include *Tieh Ta Yao Gin* (Traumatic Injury Medicine) and *Zheng Gu Shui.*

Homeopathy
Arnica (12c) may be taken every 10 minutes for one to two hours, until the shock of injury passes, and then every eight hours until the pain is gone. Taken every eight to 12 hours for up to three days, *Ruta* (12c) may aid healing after a dislocation or any tendon or ligament injury. The symptoms of any muscle strain or sprain may be eased with *Rhus toxicodendron* (12c), taken three times a day for as long as a week. For joint pain, including tennis elbow, or discomfort associated with excessive use of the

wrist, a homeopath might recommend Calcarea carbonica.

Hydrotherapy
Water is the perfect place for athletes recovering from injuries to work out. Aquatic movement provides muscle resistance without straining joints.

Lifestyle
Heat and stretching exercises before vigorous physical activity can loosen joints and soft tissue, thereby helping to prevent injury. Various types of braces and supports worn during exercise can protect joints and soft tissue and stabilize an uncomfortable joint or tendon. To avoid ankle injuries, always wear appropriate shoes with ample protection and support.

Massage
Massage can be extremely helpful in the treatment of acute traumatic injuries as well as those brought on by chronic overuse. Besides relieving aches and pains, massage shortens the recovery time after working out and helps prevent injuries. It also promotes flexibility, especially when used with stretching exercises. For serious athletes, massage helps the body cope with the wear and tear of training.

Treat a charley horse by kneading the affected area; rub in the direction of the muscle fibers.

OF SPECIAL INTEREST

Child Sports Injuries: What Parents Should Know

Each year during the high-school football season there are an estimated one million injuries; wrestling, soccer, and basketball also carry a high risk of injury.

Children are at a higher risk of injury than adult athletes because those playing together may be at vastly different weights, stages of development, and strengths. To help prevent injury, try to ensure that participants in a group are at a similar level of physical development.

Athletic Injuries

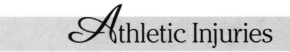
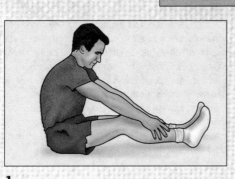

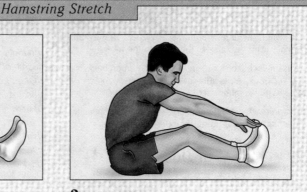

1 *Sit on the floor with your legs extended and slightly bent at the knees. Keeping your back as straight as possible, slowly bend from the hips and reach down your legs as far as you can without forcing the stretch. Hold in place for 15 seconds.*

2 *Without changing your position, reach toward your feet and try to touch your toes with your fingertips. Hold this position for 15 seconds, then slowly relax the stretch and sit back. Rest for 10 seconds, then repeat the exercise. Do eight to 10 times.*

Nutrition and Diet

Many experts advise athletes to maintain a high-carbohydrate, low-fat diet to increase energy levels and promote muscle strength.

Taken orally or topically, vitamin E may guard against muscle damage during exercise. Magnesium helps maintain muscle flexibility, which lessens susceptibility to injury.

For bone fractures, vitamin B complex and zinc may help. Nutritionists sometimes recommend supplemental use of calcium and potassium for maintenance of good musculoskeletal health.

Avoid sugar and stimulants such as caffeinated and decaffeinated beverages, particularly before exercising. Stimulants tighten muscles, increasing the risk of injury.

Home Remedies

- Replacing fluids lost through perspiration with a carbohydrate-electrolyte sports drink helps prevent cramping.
- Ice packs reduce swelling; a bag of frozen vegetables can be a makeshift ice pack. Do not use chemical cold packs, since they are much colder than water packs. Place a damp towel around your pack so that it is not directly on your skin.
- A warm compress may relieve muscle pain, especially before massage and stretching.
- To relieve cramping, elevate the affected area to direct blood flow toward the heart.
- If muscles are sore the day after a tough workout, soak in a hot tub and rest the area.

Prevention

Before you begin a sport or exercise routine, have a physical exam. This advice is particularly appropriate if you are over the age of 40.

Sports injuries usually result when the muscles are poorly conditioned. You should have a 10-minute warmup session—running in place or doing jumping jacks—before an athletic activity to increase your body temperature and diminish chances of muscle injury. Stretching after your workout will prevent soreness the next day.

Engage in your sport or exercise at least three times a week to maintain proper conditioning. ∎

B

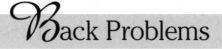

Back Problems

Symptoms

- Persistent aching or stiffness anywhere along your spine, from the base of the neck to the hips.

- Sharp, localized pain in the neck, upper back, or lower back, especially after lifting heavy objects or engaging in other strenuous activity.

- Chronic ache in the middle or lower back, especially after sitting or standing for extended periods.

Call Your Doctor If

- you feel numbness, tingling, or loss of control in your arms or legs; you may have damaged your spinal cord.

- the pain in your back extends downward along the back of the leg; you may be suffering from sciatica.

- the pain increases when you cough or bend forward at the waist; this may be the sign of a herniated disk.

- the pain is accompanied by fever; you may have a bacterial infection.

- you have dull pain in one area of your spine when lying in or getting out of bed, especially if you are over the age of 50; you may be suffering from osteoarthritis *(see Arthritis)*.

Back problems are the most common physical complaints among American adults. Non-specific back pain is a leading cause of lost job time, to say nothing of the time and money spent in search of relief. And it's all because of one characteristic that makes us different from other animals: our upright posture. Many people spend their days sitting at desks, at work stations, or in cars and trucks. Those who walk a lot or do physical labor develop good muscle tone in their backs and legs. But people who sit most of the day either lose or don't develop that muscle tone, and their backs are the first place to show it.

Treatment Options

Alternative therapies can be directed toward relieving the immediate discomfort of a back problem as well as conditioning and strengthening the body to prevent recurrence.

Acupressure
To relieve lower back pain, apply 60 seconds of thumb pressure on either side of the spine just above the top of the pelvic bone, then massage at this point, as well as at the hip and knee joints.

Acupuncture
Therapy involves inserting needles into points in specific muscles and on the ear to relieve blockages in the energy channels associated with back pain. Acute problems can be relieved in one to four sessions, while chronic pain problems typically require 12 or more treatments.

Body Work
The Alexander technique and the Feldenkrais method are useful for corrective whole-body alignment, which can relieve chronic tension and stress.

Chiropractic
Traditional chiropractic therapy relies on spinal manipulation to correct subluxations, or misaligned vertebrae, which may be responsible for problems anywhere along the spine. By helping restore motion to poorly functioning vertebrae, chiropractic therapy diminishes the accompanying pain and muscle spasm.

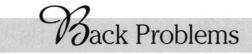

Back Problems

Herbal Therapies

For general pain relief, drink infusions of white willow (*Salix alba*) or vervain (*Verbena officinalis*). For inflammation, try teas brewed from cimicifuga (*Cimicifuga foetida*), yarrow (*Achillea millefolium*), cramp bark (*Viburnum opulus*), or white willow. Valerian (*Valeriana officinalis*) is particularly recommended as a muscle relaxant and sedative.

Homeopathy

Over-the-counter remedies reported to help non-specific back problems include *Arnica* for bruised or sore muscles, *Bryonia* and *Rhus toxicodendron* for sharp pain that gets worse when you move, and *Ruta* for persistent backache.

Massage

Muscles that parallel the spine and support it often go into spasms during attacks of back pain. Massage can reduce pain by relaxing these muscles.

Mind/Body Medicine

Biofeedback therapy is reported to help those suffering from back pain. Special electronic instruments monitor the electrical activity of the muscles, and patients learn via feedback signals how to decrease the tension or pain in their muscles.

Osteopathy

Osteopathic treatment is likely to combine drug therapy with spinal manipulation or traction, followed by physical therapy and exercise. More and more doctors and physical therapists are using spinal manipulation as part of back-pain therapy.

Yoga

Yoga postures done in a gentle way are very helpful in relaxing and stretching tense and painful muscles in the back that can lead to back problems.

Prevention

The most important preventive measure for lower back pain is practicing good posture. But it's also wise to stretch out your back if you've been sitting or standing for an hour. Analyze your posture by standing with your heels against a wall. Your

Where It Hurts

Back pain can have many causes. Pain caused by osteoarthritis (1) can occur anywhere along the spine. The larger back muscles can be affected by fibrositis (2). Pain in the loin area on

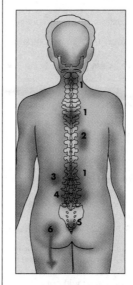

either side of the spine may indicate a kidney infection (3). Damage to spinal disks, joints, ligaments, or muscles can result in lower-back pain (4). A fall or other injury can cause pain in the coccyx (5). Pain radiating from the buttock down the back or outside of the leg may be sciatica (6).

calves, buttocks, shoulders, and the back of your head should touch the wall, and you should be able to slip your hand behind the small of your back. Then step forward and stand normally: If your posture changes, correct it right away. If you stand for long periods at work, wear flat shoes with good arch support and get a box or step about six inches high to rest one foot on from time to time.

Your sitting posture may be even more important. A good chair bottom supports your hips but doesn't touch the backs of your knees. Your chair back should be set at an angle of about 10 degrees and should cradle the small of your back comfortably; if necessary, use a wedge-shaped cushion or lumbar pad. Your feet should rest flat on the floor. Your forearms should rest on your desk or work surface with your elbows almost at a right angle. ∎

*B*ladder Infections

Symptoms

- A burning sensation when urinating; this is the most common sign of a bladder infection, but any pain or difficulty in urination may also indicate the condition.

- Frequent urge to urinate.

- Urine with a strong, foul odor.

- Heaviness or cramping in the lower abdomen.

- In the elderly: lethargy, incontinence, mental confusion.

In severe cases, these symptoms may be accompanied by fever and chills, abdominal pain, or blood in the urine. These symptoms could signal a kidney infection. See below.

Call Your Doctor If

- the burning sensation persists for more than 24 hours after you begin trying self-help treatments. Untreated, bladder infections can lead to more serious conditions.

- painful urination is accompanied by vomiting, fever, chills, bloody urine, or abdominal or back pain; it may indicate potentially life-threatening kidney disease, a kidney infection, a bladder or kidney tumor, or a prostate infection. Seek medical help immediately.

- the burning is accompanied by a discharge from the vagina or penis, a sign of sexually transmitted disease, pelvic inflammatory disease (PID), or other serious infection. See your doctor without delay.

- you experience any persistent pain or difficulty with urination; this may also be a sign of sexually transmitted disease, a vaginal infection, a kidney stone, enlargement of the prostate *(see Prostate Problems)*, or a bladder or prostate tumor. See your doctor without delay.

Bladder infections—generally termed cystitis, which means inflammation of the bladder—are common in women and very rare in men. *In fact, about half of all women get at least one bladder infection at some time in their lives. The reason may be that women have a shorter urethra, the tube that carries urine from the bladder. This relatively short passageway—only about an inch and a half long—makes it easier for bacteria to migrate into the bladder. Also, the opening to a woman's urethra lies close to both the vagina and the anus, giving bacteria from those areas access to the urinary tract. Bladder infections are not serious if treated promptly. But recurrences are common in susceptible people and can lead to kidney infections, which are more serious and may result in permanent kidney damage.*

Treatment Options

If begun promptly at the first hint of burning during urination, alternative remedies can be successful in getting rid of a bladder infection. But if these methods do not bring relief within 24 hours, you should call your doctor for antibiotic treatment. Consult with your doctor if you wish to continue with alternative methods while on the antibiotics, to speed up the recovery process.

Acupuncture

Acupuncture treatment may help prevent recurrences of bladder infections. Consult a professional acupuncturist.

Aromatherapy

Hot sitz baths can help relieve the symptoms of a bladder infection. Adding certain pungent herbal oils to the bathwater creates a soothing, fragrant steam that aromatherapists believe makes the treatment particularly effective. Try putting in a few drops of the essential oils of juniper berry, eucalyptus globulus *(E. globulus)*, sandalwood, pine, parsley, cedarwood, German chamomile *(Matricaria recutita)*, or cajuput.

You can also try a massage oil made with 1 oz vegetable oil and 5 drops each of any combination of the herbs above. Massage daily, rubbing the oil over your lower back, abdomen, stomach, and hips.

*B*ladder Infections

■ Chiropractic

Adjusting the bones and joints around the pelvis can act to strengthen the bladder muscles, helping to ward off recurrences of the infection. An osteopath can also provide this treatment.

■ Herbal Therapies

Some herbs have been found useful in both clearing up bladder infections and easing the burning that accompanies them. Perhaps the best known is cranberry, which, recent scientific studies show, has a remarkable ability to combat bladder and other urinary tract infections.

Another herb useful in treating bladder infections is nettle *(Urtica dioica),* which has anti-inflammatory properties. Mix 1 tsp dried, crushed nettle leaves or root in 1 cup boiling water. Allow the infusion to cool, then drink 1 tbsp every hour or two—up to 1 cup a day.

The evergreen shrub uva ursi *(Arctostaphylos uva-ursi),* or bearberry, which acts as a diuretic and an anti-inflammatory medication, has a long history as a folk remedy for bladder infections. Soak fresh leaves in brandy or other liquor for a few hours, then add to boiling water—about 1 tsp leaves per cup of water. If you have dried leaves, you can boil them directly in the water without a preliminary alcohol soak. Do not use uva ursi more than one week.

Women who are prone to bladder infections after sexual activity can help prevent recurrences by washing their perineal area with a medicinal solution of the herb goldenseal *(Hydrastis canadensis)* before and after intercourse. Mix 2 tsp of the herb per cup of water, bring to a boil, and simmer for 15 minutes. Cool to room temperature before using.

■ Homeopathy

- If the urge to urinate is very strong and the burning is intense, *Cantharis.*
- If you experience painful cramping with urination or your urine is very dark or bloody, *Mercurius corrosivus.*
- For women whose infections are brought on by sexual contact, *Staphysagria.*

Take these remedies every hour until symptoms disappear. If you experience no relief after 24 hours, seek professional help.

■ Nutrition and Diet

Drinking plenty of fluids to keep you urinating frequently and to flush out your urinary tract thoroughly is one of the most effective means of combating a bladder infection—whatever its cause. However, you should avoid beverages that might irritate the urinary tract and aggravate the burning. Culprits include alcohol, coffee, black tea, chocolate milk, carbonated beverages, and citrus juices. Until clear of the infection, you should also avoid potentially irritating foods such as citrus fruits, tomatoes, vinegar, sugar, chocolate, artificial sweeteners, and heavily spiced dishes. Wait 10 days after the burning is gone before reintroducing these foods and drinks—one at a time—into your diet.

Prevention

- Practice good bathroom hygiene. Clean the anal area thoroughly after a bowel movement. Women should wipe from front to back to avoid spreading fecal bacteria to the urethra.
- Urinate as soon as possible when you feel the urge, and make sure you empty your bladder completely each time.
- Drink plenty of liquids, particularly water and cranberry juice, which contains a substance that inhibits the growth of certain bacteria.

Women:
- Empty your bladder as soon as possible after intercourse to wash out any bacteria that may have been pushed into the urethra.
- Avoid using perfumed soaps, bubble baths, scented douches, and vaginal deodorants. These products contain substances that can irritate the urethra and make it more vulnerable to infection.
- If you use a diaphragm for birth control, make sure it fits properly, and don't leave it in place for too long. If you have recurring urinary tract infections, consider switching birth-control methods. ■

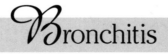ronchitis

Symptoms

Acute Bronchitis:

- Hacking cough.
- Yellow, white, or green phlegm, usually appearing 24 to 48 hours after a cough.
- Fever, chills.
- Soreness and tightness in chest.
- Some pain below breastbone during deep breathing.

Chronic Bronchitis:

- Persistent cough producing yellow, white, or green phlegm (for at least three months of the year, and for more than two consecutive years).
- Wheezing, some breathlessness.

Call Your Doctor If

- your cough is so persistent or severe that it interferes with sleep or daily activities; you could be damaging sensitive air sacs in your lungs.
- your symptoms last more than a week, and your mucus becomes darker, thicker, or increases in volume; most likely, you have an infection requiring antibiotics.
- you display symptoms of acute bronchitis and have chronic lung or heart problems or are infected with the virus that causes AIDS; respiratory infections can leave you vulnerable to more serious lung diseases, such as pneumonia.
- you have great difficulty breathing. This symptom, sometimes mistakenly associated with bronchitis, could signal asthma, emphysema, tuberculosis, heart disease, a serious allergic reaction, or cancer.

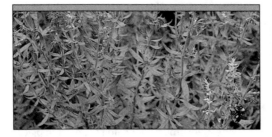

Hyssop • *To treat cases of acute bronchitis, an infusion of the herb hyssop (Hyssopus officinalis) may encourage sweating (thus lowering fever) and lessen inflammation.*

 ronchitis is an upper respiratory disease in which the mucous membrane in the upper bronchial passages becomes inflamed. As the membrane swells and grows thicker, it narrows or shuts off the tiny airways in the lungs, resulting in coughing spells accompanied by thick phlegm and breathlessness. The disease comes in two forms: acute and chronic.

Acute bronchitis sometimes accompanies an upper respiratory infection that may be either viral or bacterial. If you are otherwise in good health, the mucous membrane will return to normal after you've recovered from the initial infection, which usually lasts for several days.

Chronic bronchitis, like the lung disease emphysema, is a serious long-term disorder that requires regular medical treatment. People who have chronic bronchitis tend to be obese and lead sedentary lives, and most are heavy smokers; they typically have emphysema as well.

Treatment Options

Although acute bronchitis can often be treated effectively without a physician, you will need to see a doctor for a prescription of antibiotics if the underlying infection is bacterial. You may also benefit from a prescription cough syrup. If you suffer from chronic bronchitis, you are at risk of developing cardiovascular problems as well as more serious lung diseases and infections, so you should be monitored by a doctor.

Alternative therapies can help to ease some of the symptoms of acute and chronic bronchitis, but keep in mind that they do not always cure infections.

Aromatherapy

Essential oils such as eucalyptus globulus (*E. globulus*), hyssop (*Hyssopus officinalis*), aniseed (*Pimpinella anisum*), lavender (*Lavandula angustifolia*), pine (*Pinus sylvestris*), and rosemary (*Rosmarinus officinalis*) may help ease breathing and relieve nasal congestion. Inhaling deeply through your nose, breathe the aroma from a few drops of one or more of these oils dabbed on a handkerchief, or sniff directly from the bottle. Try mixing a few drops of essential oil in a sink full of hot water; cover your head with a towel and breathe in the fragrant steam.

*B*ronchitis

The Bronchial Tubes

Air flows down the windpipe and into the lungs through branching conduits called the bronchial tubes, or bronchioles, which normally are lined with only a thin mucous membrane. In bronchitis, however, this membrane becomes inflamed, resulting in stepped-up mucus production. Over time, excess mucus can clog the bronchioles, cutting off air flow to the lungs. Coughing is the body's way of ridding the lungs of this mucus buildup.

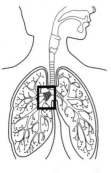

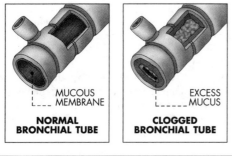

MUCOUS MEMBRANE	EXCESS MUCUS
NORMAL BRONCHIAL TUBE	**CLOGGED BRONCHIAL TUBE**

Herbal Therapies

A wide variety of herbs act as soothing expectorants. A sampling of therapies follows; for more, seek the advice of a professional herbalist.

For acute or chronic bronchitis, coltsfoot *(Tussilago farfara)* may relax bronchial tubes that are constricted or in spasm and help loosen phlegm. To prepare an infusion, add a cup of boiling water to 1 or 2 tsp coltsfoot; steep for 10 minutes. Drink it as hot as possible, three times daily. Mullein *(Verbascum thapsus),* believed to have an anti-inflammatory effect on mucous membranes, can also be prepared as an infusion according to the same directions. Expectorants appropriate for chronic bronchitis include aniseed *(Pimpinella anisum),* elecampane *(Inula helenium),* and garlic *(Allium sativum).*

Homeopathy

For acute and chronic bronchitis, take the following three times a day, for up to four days: To treat fever, cough, and tightness in the chest with anxiety, use *Aconite* (12x). For loose white phlegm, cough, and irritability, use *Kali bichromicum* (12x). For loss of voice, cough, thirst, sore throat, and exhaustion, use *Phosphorus* (12x). Consult a homeopath for the remedy that's best for you.

Nutrition and Diet

To strengthen the immune system, nutritionists often recommend vitamins A, B complex, C, and E, along with the minerals selenium and zinc. Some suggest you also avoid mucus-producing foods, found mainly in the dairy group (although goat's milk generally causes less mucus production than cow's milk) as well as in refined starches (white-flour–based products) and processed foods. ■

C

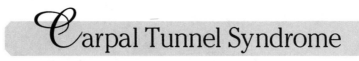
Carpal Tunnel Syndrome

Symptoms

- A tingling or numb feeling in the hand, usually just in the thumb and the first three fingers.

- Shooting pains in the wrist, forearm, and sometimes extending to the shoulder, neck, and chest.

- Difficulty clenching the fist or grasping small objects.

- Sometimes, dry skin and fingernail deterioration.

Call Your Doctor If

- the pain and numbness persist and you have not been able to find relief; your doctor can perform tests to confirm the diagnosis. Your arm and hand may have to be immobilized in a cast for several weeks, or in the worst case you may need surgery.

- you feel pain in your wrist, hand, or fingers after a fall or other accident; you may have a broken bone.

- your hands or fingers feel painful and stiff, especially if the joints become swollen; you may be suffering from a form of arthritis.

- pain in the hands and fingers is more intense at night; this may signal late-onset diabetes.

C *arpal tunnel syndrome (CTS) is one of several names for painful and disabling injuries to the thumb, fingers, and wrists, and sometimes to the elbows and other joints. As a group, these conditions are called repetitive stress injuries (RSI). The warning signs are tingling and numbness in the affected joints—typically the fingers—especially after the regular workday, or when you're ready to go to sleep, or on awakening.*

Many people think CTS came in with the computer keyboard. In fact, injuries to the carpal tunnel and other major nerve passages have been around a long time; but with so many fingers tapping away at computer keyboards, the problem is more widespread than ever. The same symptoms can develop from any repetitive manual activity, from playing sports or musical instruments to using power tools or waiting on tables. Some authorities believe that a pyridoxine (vitamin B$_6$) deficiency can also induce the symptoms.

Treatment Options

The following treatments complement the need to reduce inflammation, rest the damaged wrist, and take the necessary steps to correct the habits or activities that caused the problem in the first place.

Acupuncture
Acupuncture may provide relief by stimulating circulation, calming nerves, and releasing the body's own painkilling agents. In addition to inserting needles around the sore wrist, an experienced practitioner may treat the back, shoulders, and neck.

Chiropractic
A chiropractor will probably employ spinal adjustment of the neck and upper back to restore normal nerve activity. He or she may also manipulate the wrist, forearm, and shoulder, as well as applying a splint or brace.

Herbal Therapy
Make a soothing compress by simmering 1 to 2 oz of fresh grated ginger *(Zingiber officinale)* in 4 oz of boiling water. Dip a soft, folded cloth into the decoction and apply the hot compress to the affected area, covering it with a dry cloth to retain the heat.

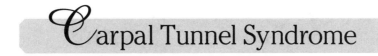 Carpal Tunnel Syndrome

Discontinue this treatment if the ginger irritates your skin or if it doesn't improve your condition.

Homeopathy

Try the following: *Arnica* (6x to 30c) for swelling and bruising caused by overuse or misuse of the joints; *Ruta* (6x to 12x) for tendon inflammation; and *Rhus toxicodendron* (6x) for pain. Or see a licensed homeopath for a more specific analysis.

Massage

Massage therapy may help in cases where pressure from soft tissues, lack of blood flow, and stress are thought to be the cause. Because CTS can involve other areas besides the wrist, massage may be used on hand, wrist, arm, shoulder, or neck areas.

Nutrition and Diet

Supplemental vitamin E in amounts up to 800 IU daily is reported to help reduce tissue inflammation. Vitamin C supplements up to 1,000 mg may be beneficial in tissue restoration. Vitamin B_6, or pyridoxine, is reported to help nerve inflammation and enhance blood circulation. Because high-protein diets inhibit the absorption of B_6, reduce your protein intake. Start with 50 mg a day, or try a vitamin B complex supplement; symptoms should ease within the month.

Osteopathy

Osteopathic physicians may recommend manipulation of the joint and surrounding soft tissue to improve circulation and nerve function.

Yoga

Yoga positions that relax the neck and back may help, but avoid hand and neck stands, as well as positions that include arm twists, any of which could harm already sensitive nerves.

Home Remedies

A few simple exercises and a cold pack may be the best treatment for reducing the discomfort of an RSI. One effective exercise is opening and closing your fist 12 or more times. Or try the following:

- With palms facing each other, press your fin-

gertips together 20 times, rest, then repeat.
- Holding your hands over your head, rotate them at the wrists clockwise for 20 seconds, then do the same exercise counterclockwise.
- Strengthen hand and forearm muscles with a spring-style or foam-rubber grip exerciser.

Prevention

The natural position of the hand in most normal activities is straight or slightly bent at the wrist, with the thumb more or less in line with the forearm. Bending the hand forward or backward at the wrist for extended periods stresses the carpal nerves, so learn to keep your wrist and hand as straight as possible when you work. Take breaks and exercise your hands and wrists every hour. If you work at a keyboard, use a wrist support to help prevent unnatural bending and make sure your desk and chair height are correct for your stature. ∎

The Wrist

The wrist is a complicated, vulnerable joint. The median nerve—which runs from the forearm to the fingertips and controls movement of the fingers and thumb—passes through a tunnel formed by carpal bones and a tough layer of ligaments. If the median nerve is stressed or pinched, your fingers feel numb or tingly and you may lose feeling in your hand.

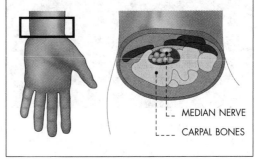

MEDIAN NERVE
CARPAL BONES

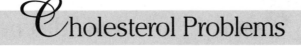

Cholesterol Problems

Symptoms

A high level of cholesterol in the blood does not have obvious symptoms but can be a risk factor for other conditions that do have recognizable symptoms, including angina, atherosclerosis, heart disease, high blood pressure, stroke, and other circulatory ailments.

■ Soft, yellowish skin growths or lesions called xanthomas may indicate a genetic predisposition to an inability to process cholesterol and triglycerides in a normal fashion.

■ Obesity and diabetes may be associated with high cholesterol levels.

■ In men, impotence may be due to arteries affected by excessive blood cholesterol.

Call Your Doctor If

■ you detect soft, yellowish skin growths on yourself or on your children. You should ask about being tested for a predisposition to high cholesterol.

■ you develop symptoms of atherosclerosis, angina, or heart disease, such as pain in the lower legs, dizziness, unsteady gait, or thick speech. Any of these conditions may be associated with high blood cholesterol, and each requires medical intervention.

Don't wait for symptoms before having your cholesterol checked. Some doctors recommend a yearly test for total blood cholesterol and for LDL- and HDL-cholesterol levels.

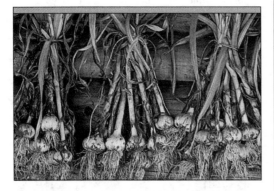

Garlic • *Members of the onion family, including garlic, may help lower your cholesterol levels, thus decreasing your risk of heart attack and stroke.*

C holesterol is a type of fat, or lipid, found in every cell of your body and is especially concentrated in your brain, liver, and blood. Cholesterol supports such vital functions as cell building, nerve insulation, hormone production, and digestion. Your body produces all the cholesterol you need. The problem is that it's easy to get too much cholesterol into your bloodstream through a fatty, high-cholesterol diet.

Every day, the average American consumes 400 to 500 mg of cholesterol in food. High cholesterol wreaks havoc on the body, increasing the risk for atherosclerosis, heart disease, and stroke.

Types of Cholesterol

In the bloodstream, cholesterol binds with protein molecules to form various types of so-called lipoproteins. Lipoproteins are classified on the basis of their protein content as high-density (more protein) or low-density (less protein). High-density lipoprotein (HDL), known as good cholesterol, is a dense, compact microparticle that transports excess cholesterol to the liver, where it is altered and expelled in the bile. Low-density lipoprotein (LDL) is a larger, less dense particle that tends to remain in the body. LDLs can deposit too much cholesterol in artery walls, impeding normal blood flow and initiating the formation of blood clots. They are an important factor in the risk for coronary heart disease—and are hence known as bad cholesterol.

Everyone has both HDLs and LDLs, but in different proportions. A higher level of HDL relative to LDL is associated with decreased risk for cholesterol problems.

Treatment Options

Alternative therapists offer a range of natural ways to control your cholesterol levels. All can be pursued independently, and many can be combined with drug therapy if your therapist considers that necessary. The following list of treatments will let you customize your own program. To be safe, advise your doctor if you are using any alternative therapeutic substances or methods before mixing them with prescription drugs.

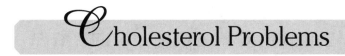

Cholesterol Problems

Ayurvedic Medicine

An Ayurvedic physician might recommend the combined formulas *Abana* and *Geriforte,* or the powder of the root *punarnava* combined with Indian bdellium. Indian bdellium's ability to control cholesterol levels has been compared with that of some synthetic drugs, with claims that it lowers LDL- and raises HDL-cholesterol levels without side effects. Indian bdellium is known as gugulipid *(Commiphora mukul)* in some Western herbal and health food stores.

Chinese Medicine

Traditional Chinese healers treat various forms of chronic heart disease, along with factors like high cholesterol, with acupuncture and an herbal therapy that employs polygonum *(Polygonum multiflorum).* Because Chinese herbs almost always work in combinations rather than individually, you should consult a trained herbalist for an appropriate prescription.

Exercise

Evidence suggests that even though exercise alone cannot lower total cholesterol, moderate exercise several times a week can help raise HDL levels in many people. Vigorous exercise may raise HDL levels even higher, although at some point athletes apparently reach an "HDL plateau."

Herbal Therapies

Herbs reputed to have cholesterol-lowering properties include alfalfa *(Medicago sativa),* turmeric *(Curcuma longa),* Asian ginseng *(Panax ginseng),* and fenugreek *(Trigonella foenum-graecum).* You might also consult a nutritionally oriented doctor about the benefits of phytosterol tablets. Phytosterols are plant compounds structurally comparable to cholesterol that effectively block uptake of cholesterol in the liver.

Nutrition and Diet

The basic dietary rules for lowering cholesterol are simple: Avoid saturated fats and dietary cholesterol. Experts recommend a high-fiber diet with not more than 30 percent of your daily calories obtained from fat; some say 20 percent. Saturated fats derived from animal products and tropical oils should be kept to a minimum, so avoid eating deep-fried foods and pay attention to nutrition labels on packaged foods. For cooking, replace saturated fats that are solid at room temperature, such as butter and shortening, with liquid monounsaturated fats such as olive, canola, or flaxseed oil. There is evidence that consuming moderate amounts of monounsaturated fat—found in such foods as nuts, seeds, and avocados—may actually lower LDL cholesterol. Eat more vegetables, fruits, and grains, which are cholesterol free and rich in fiber.

Garlic and onion are believed to lower cholesterol, but reports vary on how much you should eat in order to benefit. It's safe to say that the more you eat, preferably raw, the better the effect. Eating grapes may help reduce blood cholesterol, thanks to flavonoid compounds in their skins. Look for grape-seed oil—squeezed from grape seeds after wine pressing—for cooking and for salad dressings. Vitamins, minerals, and nutrients thought to reduce cholesterol include vitamins E, C, and A (beta carotene), L-carnitine, pantethine, chromium, calcium, copper, and zinc. To keep your menus lively, try incorporating rice bran, artichokes, shiitake mushrooms, and chili peppers—all believed to help lower cholesterol.

Select foods that contain water-soluble fiber, which offers an excellent defense against high blood cholesterol. Foods on the high-fiber list are grapefruit, apples, beans and other legumes, psyllium seed, barley, carrots, cabbage, and oatmeal.

Prevention

- Keep your weight in check.
- Eat wisely every day—no more than 300 mg of cholesterol and at the very most 30 percent of your total calories from fat.
- Exercise several times a week—vigorously if you can, but moderate exercise is better than none at all.
- Track your progress. Have your blood cholesterol level tested periodically. At-home test kits are generally unreliable.
- If you smoke, quit. ■

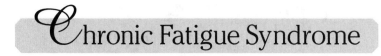

Chronic Fatigue Syndrome

Symptoms

- Recent onset of debilitating fatigue.
- Fatigue that is not a result of exertion and that is unrelieved by rest.
- Persistent low-grade fever.
- Muscle soreness and weakness.
- Sleep disorders (insomnia or oversleeping).
- Swollen, tender lymph nodes.
- Migrating joint pain without swelling or redness.
- Forgetfulness, confusion, inability to concentrate.
- Recurrent sore throat.
- Headaches.
- Long-lasting malaise following physical exertion.
- Symptoms that persist for six months and result in a substantial reduction of activities.

Call Your Doctor If

- you have overwhelming fatigue and no identifiable, obvious reason for it, such as stress. Your doctor will need to rule out other illnesses that share symptoms with chronic fatigue syndrome, such as depression, thyroid problems, mononucleosis, arthritis, lupus, and cancer.

*C*hronic fatigue syndrome, or CFS—also known as chronic fatigue and immune dysfunction syndrome (CFIDS), chronic Epstein-Barr virus (CEBV), and myalgic encephalomyelitis (ME)—first came to public attention in the mid-1980s. It primarily strikes young urban professionals, with Caucasian women under age 45 accounting for 80 percent of cases; however, anyone, even a child, is susceptible. The cause is not known, but stress may affect the immune system, leaving it susceptible to an autoimmune disorder.*

Treatment Options

A number of alternative therapies can help control the various symptoms of CFS. But be sure to check with your doctor for an accurate diagnosis before embarking on a course of treatment.

Acupuncture

An acupuncturist may undertake a series of treatments to attempt to normalize and balance the immune system. In Chinese medicine, enhancing vital energy, nourishing the blood, and strengthening the spirit can be part of the therapeutic strategy.

Herbal Therapies

Goldenseal *(Hydrastis canadensis)* has been shown to increase white blood cell activity in some tests. Echinacea *(Echinacea* spp.) and shiitake *(Lentinus edodes)* mushrooms contain oligosaccharides, known to be extremely potent immune stimulators; take in moderate doses only, as advised by a qualified herbalist. Gotu kola *(Centella asiatica)* or ginkgo *(Ginkgo biloba)* may help you to be more alert; take 10 to 15 drops of the herb, in tincture form, twice a day. There are many other herbs that may be helpful; consult with a qualified herbalist.

The Chinese herbal formula *Bu Zhong Yi Qi Wan* (Tonify the Middle and Augment the Chi Pills) is used to treat CFS; it may help boost your energy levels. Another mixture, *Xiao Chai Hu Wan* (Minor Bupleurum Pills), is especially helpful if CFS first began with flulike symptoms. A Chinese medicine practitioner may recommend a commercially prepared mixture called Astragalus Ten Formula, which combines Asian ginseng *(Panax ginseng)*, licorice *(Glycyrrhiza uralensis)*, astragalus *(Astragalus mem-*

Chronic Fatigue Syndrome

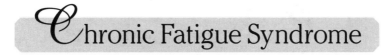

Yoga

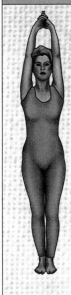

Mountain • Stress-reducing exercises may help chronic fatigue. For the Mountain, stand with your feet together. Inhale and raise your arms straight out from your sides and join them over your head. Hold for 20 seconds while breathing deeply, then exhale and slowly lower your arms. Do once or twice a day.

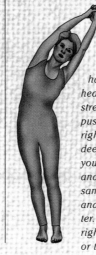

Half-Moon • To do the Half-Moon, inhale and clasp your hands over your head. Exhale and stretch to the left, pushing out your right hip. Breathe deeply, keeping your shoulders and hips on the same plane. Inhale and return to center. Repeat on the right side. Do once or twice a day.

Rag Doll • Stand with your arms at your sides, exhale, and bend forward from the waist. Let the top of your head drop toward the floor (do not force the stretch). Cup your elbows in your palms and relax, breathing deeply. Hold for 20 seconds, then inhale and slowly stand up. Do once or twice a day.

branaceus), and other herbs. Some patients report improvement after taking this formula regularly.

Mind/Body Medicine

Meditation, progressive relaxation, guided imagery, qigong, and yoga (above) may help ease CFS symptoms without being tiring. In fact, they may provide an energy boost because they reduce stress.

Nutrition and Diet

One theory holds that a nutritional deficiency may be a contributing factor causing CFS, so it's important to maintain a healthful diet. Avoid caffeine; alcohol; refined sugar; white flour; salt; and fried, preserved, high-fat foods in favor of whole grains; beans; rice; fish; and fresh fruits and vegetables. Add edible seaweeds, shiitake (Lentinus edodes) mushrooms, and licorice (Glycyrrhiza glabra) to your diet. Eating two cloves of garlic (Allium sativum) a day may help boost your immune system's antiviral and antibacterial activity.

Coenzyme Q and vitamin B_{12} are nutritional supplements that may lessen symptoms. Some evidence suggests that a combination of malic acid and magnesium may help relieve fatigue and muscle pain. Egg lecithin taken with meals may enhance immunity and promote energy. Other immune-system-enhancing vitamins are vitamin C and mixed carotenoids—including beta carotene (vitamin A). Vitamins B_5 and B_6, zinc, selenium, manganese, and chromium all play a role in strengthening the immune system as well.

Home Remedies

Make sure you don't attempt more activity than you can handle. Get plenty of rest, pay attention to your diet, and exercise lightly on a regular basis. ■

C

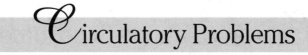

Circulatory Problems

Symptoms

- Cramplike pain, muscle fatigue, and aching in the legs; the blood vessels in your calves, thighs, feet, or hips may be blocked, possibly due to hardening of the arteries.

- Bulging, bluish vessels in an aching leg; you may have varicose veins.

- A painful vein; you may have phlebitis.

- A finger, toe, or other body part that feels numb after exposure to cold weather, then becomes red and painful once it is warmed; you could be suffering from frostbite.

Call Your Doctor If

- you experience sudden and severe localized pain, and the affected area turns pale and cold; you may have a fully blocked blood vessel, which can lead to tissue death.

- you develop skin ulcers, localized skin discoloration, or nonhealing sores; these may be signs of obstructed blood flow.

- you are experiencing pain in leg muscles while walking or resting; your blood flow may be dangerously restricted.

 ost of us experience the discomfort of tired, stiff, aching legs every now and then. Many people, however, must cope with this sensation on a daily basis. This condition, called intermittent claudication, results from blocked arteries in the pelvis, thighs, or calves and most often is caused by atherosclerosis, commonly known as hardening of the arteries.

But interruptions in normal blood flow through arteries and veins can be brought on by a variety of conditions. Weakened arterial walls, for example, can balloon out and form pockets that trap blood. Veins can stretch, causing their internal valves to malfunction, and vascular disease can cause blood vessels to constrict. Most of the time the discomfort caused by circulatory irregularities is confined to the buttocks and legs, but it can also affect other parts of the body.

Treatment Options

Many nonconventional treatments for poor circulation are attempts to strengthen weak blood vessels or widen their openings, thus allowing greater blood flow to distant parts of the body. Some alternative therapies also help to ease the discomfort or reduce the inflammation and swelling associated with circulatory problems.

Body Work
Yoga can promote blood flow and help alleviate the discomfort of poor circulation.

Chelation Therapy
Many people seek relief through chelation therapy, which involves injecting the chemical EDTA into the bloodstream. This treatment, however, is controversial and far from universally accepted.

Chinese Medicine
A traditional healer may advise a combined program of acupuncture, herbal therapy, and massage. Chinese herbs are also used in specific combinations to treat circulatory problems.

Herbal Therapies
An extract of the small, thorny hawthorn *(Crataegus laevigata)* tree promotes circulation by dilating blood vessels, particularly coronary arteries. And

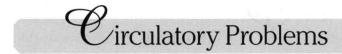

ginkgo *(Ginkgo biloba)* has a well-documented record of medicinal success. Studies show that concentrated extracts from the leaves of the ginkgo tree may help improve circulation by dilating the arteries. If you have a blood-clotting disorder, consult a doctor before using ginkgo, since the plant contains a substance thought to suppress the blood's clotting ability. Ginkgo has also been shown to cause mild side effects, including excitability and digestive problems.

Taken orally, an Asian herb called gotu kola *(Centella asiatica)* appears to benefit circulation by strengthening blood vessel walls. Cayenne *(Capsicum annuum* var. *annuum)* and ginger *(Zingiber officinale)* may stimulate circulation by dilating arterioles and capillaries near the skin's surface. Butcher's-broom *(Ruscus aculeatus)* is believed to alleviate swelling and inflammation caused by many circulatory disorders. Both cayenne and butcher's-broom also work well topically, as an oil or a lotion.

■ Hydrotherapy

A long soak in a warm bath, followed by a brisk rub with a towel dipped in cold water, can ease general discomfort brought on as a result of poor circulation. Add a decoction of thyme leaves or larch needles (larch is a type of pine) to the bathwater for a stimulating effect. Soak cold feet in a warm footbath for 15 minutes. To promote circulation in the legs, alternate hot and cold footbaths (one to two minutes in hot water, 30 seconds in cold water) for 15 minutes. WARNING: Diabetics or others with reduced temperature sensitivity in their feet or legs must use extra caution to avoid burns.

■ Massage

Massage has been proved to increase blood flow and improve circulation, and can provide some of the benefits of exercise for those unable to exercise. Avoid massaging varicose veins directly; it will damage the vessel walls and make the veins worse. People with blood clots should not have massage.

■ Neural Therapy

Intended to restore electrical conductivity in the body through injections of anesthetics, neural therapy is popular in Germany for a range of conditions, including some circulatory problems. WARNING: Neural therapy should be used only as a complement to orthodox medical treatment, not as a substitute. This technique is not recommended for patients who have cancer, diabetes, or renal failure, or for people who are allergic to local anesthetics.

■ Nutrition and Diet

As a rule, your diet should be low in fat and high in fiber. Emphasize whole grains and fresh fruits and vegetables. Avoid caffeinated drinks, since caffeine causes blood vessels to constrict. If you suffer from cold hands and feet, don't fall for the "warming" properties of hot toddies. Alcohol can make you feel warmer, but it ultimately impairs your ability to stay warm. Alcohol makes it more difficult for you to maintain your body temperature in cold weather and may even promote hypothermia.

If you suffer from hardened arteries, eat more fish. Not only is fish low in fat and high in nutritional value, but it also boosts levels of high-density lipoprotein (HDL), the "good" cholesterol that purges blood vessels of fatty deposits. For dessert, try pineapple. Studies suggest that an enzyme in pineapple called bromelain enhances circulation while reducing inflammation. Bromelain is also available as a supplement and works best if taken on an empty stomach.

■ Reflexology

Stimulate all reflex areas on the feet; the reflex areas for the adrenal glands may be particularly helpful. In addition, working the reflex areas analogous to the localized problem areas may enhance circulation.

Home Remedies

- Take regular walks or bike rides to enhance circulation in your legs. Do simple exercises, such as arm windmills, to get the blood flowing elsewhere.
- If you are taking birth-control pills, switch to another form of contraception.
- If you smoke, quit. ■

Common Cold
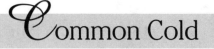

Symptoms

- Head and chest congestion, possibly with a runny nose and difficulty breathing.

- Sore throat.

- Sneezing.

- Dry cough that may occur only at night.

- Chills.

- Burning, watery eyes.

- Vague achiness all over your body.

- Headache.

Call Your Doctor If

- your newborn (two months or younger) has cold symptoms. For infants, the common cold can be a serious illness.

- congestion makes it hard for you to breathe, or your chest makes a whistling sound (a wheeze) when you breathe. You may have asthma.

- your throat hurts and your temperature is 101°F or higher; or your cold symptoms worsen after the third day. You may have a bacterial infection (such as strep throat), sinusitis, or bronchitis.

- your temperature is 103°F or higher. You may have pneumonia. Seek medical care immediately.

- your cold symptoms occur suddenly with exposure to certain triggers—such as pollen, cats, or perfume —and/or the symptoms continue for weeks. You probably have an allergy.

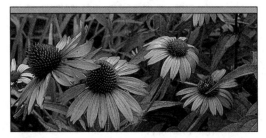

Echinacea • *A popular garden perennial, the herb echinacea contains ingredients that may help the body fight organisms such as those responsible for the common cold.*

The aptly named common cold is the most frequent infection in all age groups in the United States. Cold symptoms are triggered when a virus attaches itself to the lining of your nasal passages or throat. Your immune system responds by attacking the germ with white blood cells called neutrophils. If your immune system cannot recognize the virus, the response is "nonspecific," meaning your body produces as many neutrophils as possible (usually more than are needed) and circulates them to the infected sites. This all-out attack kills many viruses, but it doesn't affect the 200 or so viruses that cause colds. Extra neutrophils clumping together at infection sites are what cause the achiness and inflammation of a cold, complete with vast amounts of mucus in the nose and throat.

Cold symptoms begin between one and four days after you are infected by a cold virus and typically last for about three days. During the time you have symptoms, you are contagious (meaning you can pass the cold to others). The illness usually goes away in a week or so without any special medicine.

Treatment Options

Begin to treat your cold as soon as you feel the first symptom. Especially with herbal remedies, an early response often results in a faster and easier recovery. (Pregnant or nursing mothers should check with their doctor before using herbal remedies.)

Aromatherapy
Herbal steam can reduce congestion, and if the vapor temperature is 110°F or higher, it will also kill cold germs on contact. Choose eucalyptus globulus *(E. globulus),* wintergreen *(Gaultheria procumbens),* or peppermint *(Mentha piperita).* Place fresh leaves in a bowl and pour in boiling water. Place a towel over your head, lean over the bowl to create a steam tent, and breathe the vapors.

Herbal Therapies
Taken at the first sign of symptoms, echinacea *(Echinacea* spp.) can reduce a cold's intensity and duration, often even preventing it from becoming a full-fledged infection. Echinacea apparently stimulates the immune response, enhancing resistance to all infection. It is most palatable in capsules and

Common Cold

tincture. Goldenseal *(Hydrastis canadensis)* helps clear mucus from the throat. It also contains the natural antibiotic berberine, which can help prevent bacterial infections that often follow colds. Take 10 to 15 drops of either herb in an alcohol-free form, known as glycerite tincture, two to three times a day for seven to 10 days.

For a good "cold tea," combine equal parts elder *(Sambucus nigra),* peppermint *(Mentha piperita),* and yarrow *(Achillea millefolium)* and steep 1 to 2 tsp of the mixture in 1 cup hot water. This blend can help the body handle fever and reduce achiness, congestion, and inflammation.

Garlic *(Allium sativum)* appears to shorten a cold's duration and severity. Any form seems to work: capsules or tablets, oil rubbed on the skin, or whole garlic roasted or cooked in other foods. If you elect capsules, take three of them, three times daily, until the cold is over.

The Chinese herbal formula *Yin Qiao Pian* is said to be very effective for stopping a cold at the outset. *Sang Ju Yin Pian* (Mulberry Chrysanthemum Pills) is another cold remedy.

▇ Homeopathy

Cold symptoms often respond well to homeopathic remedies. The dosage is 12c, taken every two hours for a maximum of four doses. *Gelsemium* may help if you have chills, aching arms and legs, and fatigue, or if your throat hurts. When your runny nose feels as though it burns, your eyes water constantly, and you sneeze often, try *Allium cepa.* If you feel irritable and have a runny nose that becomes congested at night, take *Nux vomica.* For a barking cough, a burning sore throat, and a bitter taste that lingers in your mouth, try *Aconite.* To prevent a cold, take one dose *Ferrum phosphoricum* (6x) every morning during cold season.

▇ Lifestyle

Refrain from smoking, especially when you have a cold. Smoking assaults the mucous membranes and lungs, increasing your susceptibility to all sorts of respiratory infections, including colds. Once you have a cold, smoke irritates the already-inflamed tissues, making healing and recovery more difficult.

▇ Nutrition and Diet

Good nutrition is essential for resisting and recovering from a cold. Eat a balanced diet. Take supplements as needed to ensure you are receiving the recommended dietary allowances for vitamin A, the vitamin B complex *(vitamins B_1, B_2, B_5, B_6, folic acid),* and vitamin C, as well as the minerals zinc and copper. If your diet is deficient in zinc, your body is low in neutrophils, and you're an easy mark for all types of infections, including colds. Zinc is available as a tablet or throat lozenge. While you have a cold, avoid dairy products, which tend to make mucus thicker. You also should avoid caffeinated and decaffeinated beverages and white sugar, which weaken the immune system.

"Jewish penicillin," also known as chicken soup, has been heralded as a cold therapy since the 12th century. Recent scientific evidence supports the notion that the soup reduces cold symptoms, especially congestion. Something (yet to be determined) in the chicken soup keeps neutrophils from clumping together and causing inflammation.

Any food spicy enough to make your eyes water will have the same effect on your nose, promoting drainage. If you feel like eating, a hot, spicy choice will help your body fight your cold.

Home Remedies

- Get plenty of rest. You may find you need 12 hours or more of sleep per night while you're fighting a cold.
- Keep your body hydrated by drinking up to eight glasses of fluid each day; this will replace the fluids lost through perspiration and your runny nose and minimize congestion.

Prevention

A strong immune system is the best defense against all infections. Boost your body's natural resistance by eating well, not smoking, and drinking plenty of fluids every day. Minimize contact with people who have colds, or at least don't share towels, silverware, or beverages with them. Cold viruses often survive for hours on doorknobs, money, and other surfaces, so wash your hands frequently. ■

C

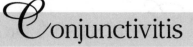

Conjunctivitis

Symptoms

- Burning, itchy eyes that discharge a heavy, sticky mucus may indicate bacterial conjunctivitis, commonly known as pinkeye.

- Copious tears, a swollen lymph node, and a light discharge of mucus from one eye are signs of viral conjunctivitis.

- Redness, intense itching, tears in the eyes, and sometimes an itchy, runny nose may indicate allergic conjunctivitis.

Call Your Doctor If

- you physically injure your eye. Eye injuries can become infected and lead to corneal ulcers, which can endanger your eyesight.

- your eyes become red when you wear contact lenses. Remove the lenses immediately and see your ophthalmologist; you may have a corneal infection.

- the redness in your eye affects your vision and is accompanied by severe pain or an excessive yellow or green discharge. You may have a staph infection or a streptococcal infection.

- your conjunctivitis frequently recurs or appears to be getting worse after a week of home treatment; you may have a bacterial or viral infection.

- your newborn baby's eyes are inflamed and are not producing tears; this may indicate a form of conjunctivitis known as ophthalmia neonatorum, which must be treated immediately by a physician to prevent permanent eye damage.

T*he conjunctiva—the transparent membrane that lines your eyeball and your eyelid—can become inflamed for various reasons. Conjunctivitis is caused by a bacterial or viral infection or by an allergic reaction to pollen, smoke, or other material that irritates your eyes. In most cases, the inflammation clears up in a few days. Although conjunctivitis can be highly contagious, it is rarely serious and will not damage your vision if detected and treated promptly.*

Bacterial conjunctivitis, commonly known as pinkeye, usually infects both eyes and produces a heavy discharge of mucus. Viral conjunctivitis is usually limited to one eye, causing copious tears and a light discharge. Allergic conjunctivitis produces tears, itching, and redness in the eyes, and sometimes an itchy, runny nose.

Ophthalmia neonatorum is an acute form of conjunctivitis in newborn babies. It must be treated immediately by a physician to prevent permanent eye damage or blindness.

Treatment Options

Alternative therapies rely on natural remedies in order to soothe irritated eyes and ease the itching and inflammation.

Aromatherapy

Myrtle hydrosol (myrtle water) will ease eye inflammation. Put it into a sterile spray bottle and carefully direct a light spray at the eyes.

Ayurvedic Medicine

An Ayurvedic physician may recommend an eyewash made from the root of barberry, the fruit rind of pomegranate, or the flower of jasmine.

Chinese Medicine

A qualified practitioner of Chinese medicine can prescribe a regimen of acupuncture or an herbal remedy such as *Niu Huang Shang Qing Wan* (Calculus Bovis Clear the Upper Pills).

Herbal Therapies

Using an eyecup, wash the eye several times a day with one of the following solutions. In each case, cool and strain the eyewash through a sterile cloth before using.

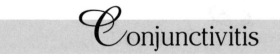

- 1 tsp dried eyebright *(Euphrasia officinalis)* steeped in 1 pt boiling water.
- 2 to 3 tsp chamomile *(Matricaria recutita)* in 1 pt boiling water.

Homeopathy

Depending on your symptoms, take the following remedies four times daily for one or two days:

- for stinging eyes and red, puffy eyelids that are relieved by cold compresses, *Apis* 12x.
- for bloodshot eyes, sharp, splinterlike pains, and a gritty feeling, *Argentum nitricum* 12x.
- for itchy eyes with a sticky, yellow discharge, *Pulsatilla* 12x.

Hydrotherapy

Place an ice-cold compress on your eyes for 20 minutes, alternating eyes every two or three minutes. Stop for 30 minutes or an hour, then reapply for 20 minutes. If only one eye is infected, treat it two minutes on, two minutes off; don't use the same compress on the healthy eye because you might spread the infection. Or try placing a hot compress over each eye for one to five minutes, followed by a potato poultice—made of grated raw potato wrapped in a porous cotton or muslin cloth—covered with a cold washcloth.

For chronic conjunctivitis, alternate hot and cold compresses—three minutes hot, one minute cold—repeated four times. Finish with cold.

Home Remedies

You can cleanse and soothe irritated eyes with a prepared boric acid eyewash, or try the herbal eyewashes above. To relieve the discomfort of bacterial or viral conjunctivitis, apply a warm compress for five to 10 minutes, three to four times a day. For allergic conjunctivitis, place a cool compress or a cool, moist tea bag on your closed eye. If the condition does not improve in five days, consult an ophthalmologist.

Prevention

Bacterial and viral conjunctivitis are highly contagious. Unless you take preventive measures, the condition may spread to your other eye or to other people.

- Wash your hands often and well.
- Keep your hands away from the infected eye.
- Do not share washcloths, towels, pillowcases, or handkerchiefs with other family members.
- Change your washcloth, towel, and pillowcase after each use, and wash them thoroughly.
- Do not use other people's eye cosmetics, particularly eye pencils and mascara.

If your child gets pinkeye, you should keep him or her out of school for a few days. It is not uncommon for conjunctivitis to spread from one student to an entire class. ∎

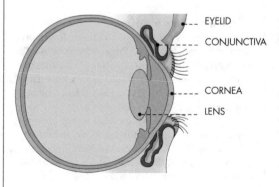

EYELID

CONJUNCTIVA

CORNEA

LENS

A Protective Layer

The conjunctiva is a thin, protective membrane that covers the exposed white of the eye and the inside of the eyelid. Bacterial conjunctivitis— sometimes called pinkeye—is the result of an infection that makes the conjunctiva red, teary, and itchy, with a thick greenish yellow discharge. When conjunctivitis is caused by an allergy, the discharge is clear and watery.

Constipation

Symptoms

- Hard, compacted stools that are difficult or painful to pass.

- No bowel movements in three days for adults, four days for children.

Call Your Doctor If

- your constipation is associated with fever and lower abdominal pain, and your stools are thin or loose; these symptoms may be an indication of diverticulitis.

- you have blood in your stools; this may be from a fissure or a hemorrhoid but could also be a sign of colorectal cancer; changes in your bowel movement pattern, such as passing pencil-thin stools, may also signal colorectal cancer.

- your constipation develops after you start a new prescription drug or take vitamin or mineral supplements; you may need to discontinue use or change the dosage.

- you or your child has been constipated for two weeks, with recurrent abdominal pain; this could be a sign of lead poisoning or another serious ailment.

- you are elderly or disabled and have been constipated for a week or more; you may have an impacted stool.

Yoga

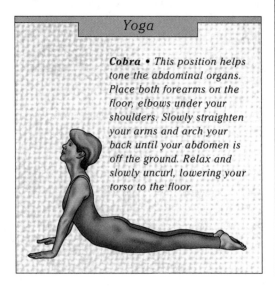

Cobra • *This position helps tone the abdominal organs. Place both forearms on the floor, elbows under your shoulders. Slowly straighten your arms and arch your back until your abdomen is off the ground. Relax and slowly uncurl, lowering your torso to the floor.*

Y*our digestive system is remarkably efficient: In the space of a few hours it extracts nutrients from the foods you eat and drink, processes them into the bloodstream, and prepares leftover material for disposal. That material passes through 20 or more feet of intestine before being stored temporarily in the colon, where water is removed. The residue is excreted through the bowels, normally within a day or two.*

Some people—including many alternative therapists—say we should move our bowels one to three times a day to remain healthy, but this remains controversial. Regularity very much depends on your diet, your age, and your daily activity. Nonetheless, the longer fecal material sits in the colon, the harder the stool becomes and the more difficult it is to pass. A normal stool should not be either unusually hard or soft, and you shouldn't have to strain unreasonably to pass it.

Our busy modern lifestyles may be responsible for most cases of constipation: not eating enough fiber or drinking enough water, not getting enough exercise, and not taking the time to respond to an unmistakable urge to defecate. Emotional and psychological problems can also lead to constipation.

Treatment Options

Most health professionals approach constipation as a lifestyle problem. Corrective measures include increasing fiber consumption, exercising regularly, and setting a routine time to move your bowels. You should seek the advice of a doctor if your problem is chronic or severe.

■ Acupressure

Digestion may be improved by steady finger pressure on Stomach 36, four finger widths below the kneecap just outside the shinbone. Maintain pressure for one minute, then switch legs. To verify the location, flex your foot; you should feel a muscle bulge at the point site. *(See page 67.)*

As an aid to relieving constipation, try applying pressure to Large Intestine 11, on the outer edge of the inside elbow crease. With the arm bent, press deeply into the point with your thumb for one minute, then repeat on the other arm. *(See page 49.)*

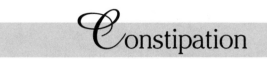

Constipation

Exercise

Walking for 20 to 30 minutes at a pace fast enough to get the heart pumping, or a good session at some other exercise, helps stimulate the bowels. Doctors say regular exercise, besides offering cardiac benefits, is an excellent way to correct chronic constipation. People should become accustomed to regular exercise when they are young so that it becomes a healthy, lifelong habit.

Herbal Therapies

Your health food store will have a selection of potentially useful herbal remedies. Try small amounts to test the effect they have on you or take them as recommended by a naturopath. Avoid herbal laxatives containing senna *(Cassia senna)* or buckthorn *(Rhamnus purshiana);* they can damage the lining and injure the nerves of the colon, and you can become dependent on them.

Homeopathy

For relief of mild constipation, you can find prepared remedies at a health food store. If your stools are soft but you have to strain to pass them, try remedies containing *Bryonia.*

Lifestyle

Simply recognizing the need to move the bowels solves many cases of constipation. Children respond to praise for sitting on the toilet and having regular bowel movements, and they can be trained at an early age.

For people who are convinced that regular bowel habits are important, the treatment is simple: Sit on the toilet every day at the same time for about 10 minutes, even if you don't have an urge to move your bowels. The best time is after a meal, because food in the stomach stimulates the colon to move. Be patient: It may take a couple of months before this new habit begins to work for you. Remember, however, to heed your body's own signals and to never resist the urge to move your bowels at other times.

Nutrition and Diet

Almost all Americans should eat more fiber. The American Dietetic Association recommends 30 grams of fiber a day, yet many people consume less than half that amount. Increasing your fiber intake is easy: Eat more raw fruits and vegetables—especially peas, beans, and broccoli—bran cereals, whole-wheat bread, and dried fruits such as raisins, figs, and prunes. A bonus is that most of these foods are rich in vitamins and minerals yet lower in calories than most processed foods.

It is never too early to start a healthy diet. Children as young as six months can be fed whole-grain cereals, which have more fiber and more nutrients than processed cereals. Even fast-food addicts can be tempted into snacking on fruit and raw vegetables. Otherwise, try a soluble or insoluble fiber supplement like psyllium *(Plantago psyllium),* which becomes gelatinous when combined with water and adds bulk to the stool. Drink 1 to 2 rounded tsp of powdered psyllium a day, stirred into a glass of cold water or juice, or include an equal amount of powdered flaxseed *(Linum usitatissimum),* available in many health food stores. Psyllium generally works within two days, but you can take it every day and not become dependent on it.

Insoluble fibers, including wheat bran, work as well as psyllium but may give you gas for a few weeks until your system adjusts to the change. You can mix bran with fruit juice, canned fruit, or cereal, or sprinkle it into sandwiches. Start by taking 1 tbsp a day, and gradually increase it to 3 or 4 spoonfuls.

An old folk remedy for stimulating the bowels is to drink a glass of warm water containing the juice of a whole lemon after waking in the morning and 15 minutes before each meal.

Prevention

The key to preventing constipation is simple: Drink adequate amounts of water—six to eight glasses a day is a good rule—and get sufficient fiber by eating fruits, vegetables, and grains. Fiber is critical because a large proportion of our stool is made up of bacteria, and fiber gives bacteria a good foundation to grow on. Ample bacterial action results in a larger volume of stool and better bowel function. ∎

C

Cough

Symptoms

More important than the cough itself are aspects of it that provide clues to its cause:

- Frequency and duration of the cough.

- Length of the coughing spell.

- Type of material being coughed up (mucus or phlegm, blood).

- Color of the sputum (white, clear, green, yellow, pink, blood-specked).

- Consistency of the material coughed up (thick, thin, frothy).

- Presence or absence of accompanying pain.

Call Your Doctor If

- your cough lasts for more than seven to 10 days; it may be a sign of a serious disease.

- your cough is producing yellow, green, pink, or rust-colored sputum.

- your cough is exhausting, persistent, and accompanied by any of the following signs: hoarseness, sore throat, shortness of breath, wheezing, chest pains or tightness, fever of 101°F or higher, headache, back and leg aches, fatigue, rashes, or weight loss. A cough combined with one or more of these symptoms indicates an underlying ailment.

A lthough it is usually unwelcome and involuntary, a cough is not itself an illness but rather a protective reflex. Generally, the reflex kicks in when the membranes lining the respiratory tract secrete excessive mucus or phlegm. These secretions help to protect your airways from infections and irritants by trapping and flushing out viruses, bacteria, and foreign particles. Coughing is your body's way of getting rid of this accumulation. The sudden burst of air in a cough not only helps to keep the breathing passages open but also helps to clear the lungs and bronchial tubes. But be aware that severe coughing could indicate such serious infections as pneumonia or bronchitis.

Treatment Options

Most coughs are not dangerous. Therefore, if you have a nonproductive (dry) cough accompanied by a runny or stuffed-up nose, a sore throat, and sneezing, you have all the classic symptoms of a common cold, and you should just let it run its course.

The following therapies may ease the discomfort of an acute or chronic respiratory infection, but they will not treat the infection itself. It's best to use cough remedies for no longer than seven to 10 days and preferably only for temporary relief from nighttime coughing.

Acupressure

Sometimes a coughing fit can make the muscles in the upper back contract or go into spasm. To relieve the pain this causes, apply pressure to Lung 5 (opposite).

Herbal Therapies

A wide variety of herbs act as stimulating or relaxing expectorants that help the body remove excess mucus from the airways. Stimulating expectorants increase the quantity of and then liquefy viscous sputum so it can be cleared out by coughing. Relaxing expectorants loosen the sputum and are soothing if you have a dry, irritating cough.

Since most herbal traditions have remedies for specific types of coughs, you might want to check the many possibilities with an herbalist. However, a basic herbal tea for cough that can be

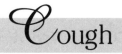 Cough

taken several times a day for three days consists of 2 parts coltsfoot *(Tussilago farfara)*, 2 parts marsh mallow *(Althaea officinalis)*, 2 parts hyssop *(Hyssopus officinalis)*, 1 part aniseed *(Pimpinella anisum)*, and 1 part licorice *(Glycyrrhiza glabra)*. Add to 1 cup boiling water, steep for 20 minutes, and drink while hot.

There are many good Chinese herbal cough medicines available in Asian food stores. Among them are Fritillaria and Loquat Cough Mixture, King To's Natural Herb Loquat Flavored Syrup, and *San She Dan Chuan Bei Ye.*

Homeopathy

Homeopaths recommend different remedies and dosage schedules for the beginning and later stages of various types of coughs. For relief of early symptoms, take one dose four times a day; for relief of persistent symptoms, take one dose twice a day for four days. If a dry cough comes on suddenly with fever and restlessness, try *Aconite* (12c). If you are often thirsty and have painful bouts of dry coughs that intensify with the slightest movement, try *Bryonia* (12c). If your throat tickles and you get violent coughing fits whenever you lie down, try *Drosera* (12c). If the slightest draft of cool air initiates a tickling cough, take *Rumex crispus* (12c). If your cough is accompanied by hoarseness, difficulty in breathing, and considerable rattling in the chest, take *Antimonium tartaricum* (12c), which is particularly good for a well-established, productive cough.

Nutrition and Diet

The best thing to do for a cough is to drink plenty of liquids; usually this means four to six large glasses a day. A large intake of fluids will loosen the mucus and make coughing it up easier. Warm liquids, or just plain water, are best for this purpose. Try to avoid caffeinated or alcoholic beverages, which are diuretics that cause you to lose more liquid than you take in.

Most health professionals agree that you might speed recovery by drinking fresh fruit and vegetable juices. Some practitioners recommend vitamin C supplements; others consider a well-balanced diet just as effective.

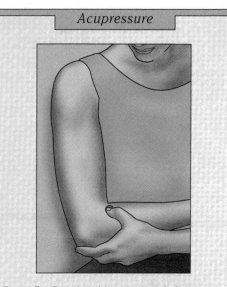

Acupressure

Lung 5 • *Pressing this point may help ease coughing spasms. Bend your right elbow and make a fist; place your left thumb on the outside crease of the elbow alongside the taut tendon. Press firmly for one minute, and repeat on the other arm. Do three times.*

Home Remedies

Besides drinking plenty of liquids, including herbal teas, rubbing your throat and chest with essential oil of eucalyptus globulus *(E. globulus)* or myrrh *(Commiphora molmol)* may give you relief. A simple rub might help you breathe more easily, cough less, and get a good night's sleep.

Another way to reduce persistent night coughing is to sleep with the head of your bed raised six to eight inches. This prevents the pooling of secretions and the return of the irritating acidic contents from your stomach to your esophagus, which you may be breathing in *(see Sore Throat)*. Try to avoid caffeine and peppermint.

You can make an effective expectorant with organic honey and a large onion. Slice the onion into rings, place in a deep bowl, cover with honey, and let stand 10 to 12 hours. Strain and take a tablespoon of this mixture four or five times a day. ■

Depression
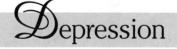

Symptoms

With major depression, you may experience four or more of the following:

- Persistent sadness, pessimism.
- Feelings of worthlessness, helplessness, hopelessness, or guilt.
- Loss of interest or pleasure in usual activities, including sex.
- Difficulty concentrating.
- Insomnia or oversleeping.
- Weight gain or loss.
- Fatigue, lack of energy.
- Anxiety, agitation, irritability.
- Thoughts of suicide or death.
- Slow speech; slow movements.

In children and adolescents:

- Insomnia, fatigue, headache, stomachache, dizziness.
- Apathy, social withdrawal, weight gain or loss.
- Drug or alcohol abuse, a drop in school performance, difficulty concentrating.
- Isolation from family and friends.

For dysthymia (minor but chronic depression), your symptoms will be less intense, fewer in number, but longer lasting.

Call Your Doctor If

- you or your child has suicidal thoughts, or has other signs of either major depression or dysthymia; professional help is available.

CAUTION

There is a distinct difference between feeling "depressed" and having a depressive illness. If you have low spirits for a while, don't be concerned. However, if you feel you can't lift yourself out of your misery, you should seek professional help.

A lmost all of us feel low sometimes, usually because of a disturbing event in our lives. But ongoing depression—or suffering a period of what is known as major depression—is a serious condition that can lead to an inability to function or may even lead to suicide. Sufferers experience not only a depressed mood but also more harmful symptoms, including lack of interest in their usual activities, extreme fatigue, sleep problems, or feelings of guilt and helplessness. They are more likely to lose touch with reality, occasionally even having delusions or hallucinations.

Major depression often goes undiagnosed because it is confused with the normal low feelings that may arise because of a specific life situation. Also of concern is minor but chronic depression, also known as dysthymia, which can last two years or more. Although the exact causes are unknown, researchers currently believe that both forms are caused by a malfunction of the brain's neurotransmitters, chemicals (particularly norepinephrine and serotonin) that modulate moods.

Treatment Options

Treatment for depression varies according to the cause of the condition and its severity. Conventional methods include psychotherapy, antidepressant drugs, and electroconvulsive therapy. Alternative therapies are particularly effective for minor depression, but for more serious depressions they should be considered as complementary treatments, not replacements for conventional methods. Major or chronic depression should be treated by a psychiatrist.

In addition to the remedies mentioned below, you may want to consider acupressure or acupuncture, which may be helpful in relieving some symptoms; see a qualified, experienced practitioner. Massage, which is both soothing and energizing and enlivens the body, may also help. Try it once a week, if possible.

Aromatherapy

Aromatherapy may ease mental fatigue and help with sleep. The essential oils that may benefit depression are basil, clary sage *(Salvia sclarea)*, jasmine, rose, and German chamomile *(Matricaria recutita)*. The oil may be placed in a bowl of steaming

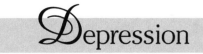

Depression

water (2 or 3 drops), in a bath (5 or 6 drops), or on the edge of your pillow (1 or 2 drops).

Exercise

Physical activity should be a part of any therapy for depression; it improves blood flow to the brain, elevates mood, and relieves stress. Even if used alone, exercise can often bring startling results. Studies show that jogging for 30 minutes three times a week can be as effective as psychotherapy in treating depression. Pick an exercise you like and do it daily, if possible. Any exercise is fine; the more energetic and aerobic, the better.

Herbal Therapies

An experienced herbalist will recommend a particular combination of herbs tailored to your specific symptoms. For a general prescription for depression, one suggestion is 2 parts St.-John's-wort *(Hypericum perforatum),* 1 part oat *(Avena sativa)* straw, 1 part lavender *(Lavandula officinalis),* and 1 part mugwort *(Artemisia vulgaris)* leaf. Take 5 ml of the tincture three times a day for at least one month. St.-John's-wort, taken in any of its forms, is a traditional depression remedy in Europe. However, some herbalists report that its effects are unpredictable: Sometimes the herb gets remarkable results, other times it has no effect at all.

A combination of several Chinese and Western herbs known as Aspiration is believed to help lift depression. The formula addresses physical symptoms as well as psychological ones, including loss of appetite, chest constriction, and constipation. It is most effective when taken in conjunction with regular aerobic exercise, daily practice of a relaxation technique, and a good diet. Another Chinese herbal formula, Gather Vitality, may help with insomnia or oversleeping, aching limbs, and fatigue. Consult a practitioner of Chinese medicine.

Mind/Body Medicine

Many mind/body practices are helpful with depression. Music and dance can lift the spirits and energize the body. Meditation and relaxation techniques, such as progressive muscle relaxation, both stimulate and relax. Other choices include transcendental meditation and the exercise tech-niques of yoga, t'ai chi, and qigong. Choose one or two that suit you and practice daily.

Anecdotal evidence suggests that EEG (brain-wave) biofeedback is effective in reducing the intensity of all types of depression. The number of training sessions depends on the severity of the depression; dysthymia may average 20 sessions, and major depression may need 30 to 60.

Nutrition and Diet

Because depressive symptoms are exacerbated by nutritional deficiencies, good nutrition is important. Increase your intake of healthful foods such as whole-grain cereals, lean meats, fruits and vegetables, fish, and low-fat dairy products. It's very important to avoid alcohol, but also stay away from junk food, sugar, aspartame, and caffeine, which give you a sudden spurt of energy or a high feeling but then bring you down.

Recent clinical studies strongly suggest that vitamin B complex and folic acid (400 mcg daily) are useful in treating depression. The antioxidant selenium (100 mcg daily) was shown to have a mood-elevating effect when taken in regions where food is deficient in selenium. And many European studies show that the amino acid supplement L-tryptophan, known to increase the synthesis of serotonin, is of value in relieving depression. Although L-tryptophan, which is the amino acid tryptophan in its synthetic form, is no longer available in the U.S., tryptophan can be found in certain foods, such as milk, turkey, chicken, fish, cooked dried beans and peas, brewer's yeast, peanut butter, nuts, and soybeans. Eat plenty of these foods together with a carbohydrate (potatoes, pasta, rice), which will ease the brain's uptake of tryptophan.

Prevention

Some forms of depression may not be preventable, since current theory suggests that they may be triggered by neurochemical malfunctioning in the brain. However, there is good evidence that a low mood may often be alleviated or prevented by good health habits. Proper diet, exercise, vacations, no overwork, and making time to do things you enjoy all help keep the blues at bay. ∎

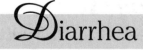 Diarrhea

Symptoms

- Frequent or watery stools, possibly with abdominal cramping, may be a result of overeating fiber-rich foods or drinking too much coffee.

- Recurrent stools with mucus, possibly accompanied by lower abdominal pain that worsens with eating or stress; you may have irritable bowel syndrome.

- A sudden attack of frequent, watery stools that may be bloody, possibly accompanied by nausea, fever, and abdominal cramping. You may have a case of gastroenteritis.

Call Your Doctor If

- you have recurrent, foul-smelling stools that are pale or yellowish; stomach cramps; weakness. These are signs of malabsorption.

- you have watery bowel movements accompanied by nervousness, insomnia, or excessive sweating. You may have diabetes or a thyroid problem.

- you have loose stools, possibly with visible blood; these are signs of various disorders, including colorectal cancer.

- you have episodes of frequent, watery stools accompanied by coughing, wheezing, and a flushed face; these symptoms may be an indication of a carcinoid tumor (a growth in the intestine that could be benign or malignant).

- you have watery stools that may be black; abdominal pain; and possibly, bright red bleeding; you could have diverticulitis. Call your doctor today to obtain a proper diagnosis.

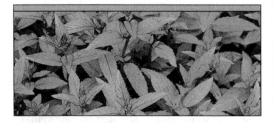

Peppermint • *Peppermint's medicinal value comes from its primary chemical constituent, menthol, a natural anti-spasmodic. A cup of peppermint tea helps to relax the muscles lining the digestive tract, thereby relieving the spasms that may accompany diarrhea.*

Diarrhea, a general term used to describe the frequent passage of loose, watery stools, is the body's way of cleaning out the digestive system—a process that usually occurs with unpleasant efficiency and some abdominal pain. Not many people make it through life without suffering at least one or two bouts of diarrhea.

Technically speaking, diarrhea is not a disease itself but rather a symptom of some other problem. The culprit can be as simple as a spicy meal or as serious as colorectal cancer. One of the most common forms is traveler's diarrhea, a variety of gastroenteritis brought on by the ingestion of food or water that has been contaminated by microorganisms as a result of improper handling. Many North Americans who have visited Latin America, the Middle East, Africa, or Asia are all too familiar with this condition, which is marked by four or five watery stools per day, abdominal cramps, nausea, and fever.

Stress or depression can lead to a type known as emotion-induced diarrhea. Diarrhea can also be caused by malabsorption—a digestive disorder in which fats and nutrients are not properly absorbed by the intestines—or by any number of other conditions, including diverticulitis, Crohn's disease, colitis, and diabetes.

In most cases of diarrhea, symptoms clear up within a few days. However, if your pain is severe or prolonged; if your stool contains blood, pus, or mucus; or if you show signs of dehydration (constant thirst, sunken eyeballs, dry lips), you should see a doctor immediately.

Treatment Options

Ayurvedic Medicine
An Ayurvedic physician may recommend a combined formula such as *Diarex* or *Bonnisan*, depending on the nature of the problem. Acute diarrhea may respond to a blending of equal parts yogurt and water with ⅛ tsp of fresh ginger. Chronic cases may respond to a powder of the fruit of beleric myrobalan.

Chinese Medicine
Many people find relief from diarrhea through acupuncture and specific combinations of Chinese herbs. Consult a qualified practitioner for treatment tailored to your specific needs.

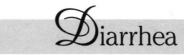 Diarrhea

Exercise

Stress can bring on a case of diarrhea or contribute to its intensity. Regular physical activity helps reduce stress.

Herbal Therapies

Taken three times daily, peppermint *(Mentha piperita)* or chamomile *(Matricaria recutita)* tea may ease intestinal spasms and cramps. You can also buy aloe vera juice: Sip half a cup slowly, twice a day.

Homeopathy

Several homeopathic remedies are used to treat diarrhea; you can choose a remedy by the accompanying symptoms:

- For burning pain when passing stools, *Arsenicum album* (12x).
- For abdominal pain, *Colocynthis* (12x).
- For watery, painless stools, *Phosphorus* (12x).

Hydrotherapy

Practitioners rely on a variety of hydrotherapy techniques for treating diarrhea. These include a heating compress to the abdomen and a 15-minute hot fomentation twice daily. Charcoal capsules are also used: Take two capsules with eight ounces of water after each bout of diarrhea.

Another common remedy is a hot half bath: After a bath in very warm water followed by a cold friction rub or shower, you are put in bed, wrapped in blankets, and allowed to sweat for 30 minutes to an hour. During the procedure, the practitioner monitors your temperature and makes sure you have plenty of water to drink.

Massage

Administered by a skilled practitioner, gentle massage to the midsection of the body can help improve intestinal activity and soothe the discomfort of diarrhea.

Nutrition and Diet

The best advice for diarrhea sufferers is to drink plenty of clear liquids, even if you're not thirsty. Slightly salty or sweet drinks—broths, sweetened tea, ginger ale, and soda, for example—are particularly helpful. Stay away from citrus drinks and milk or milk products. Also avoid foods that are high in fiber, such as grains and most fruits. When your condition starts to improve, ease your way back into a normal diet by concentrating on foods that are easily digestible, such as bland cereal, gelatin, soft-boiled eggs, white rice, applesauce, and cooked carrots.

To help replace vital stores of potassium lost to diarrhea, many nutritionists recommend ripe bananas. You can make your own nourishing potassium broth at home. In a big pot of water, simmer 2 cups chopped carrots and 2 cups chopped potatoes for 45 minutes. Drink 2 to 3 cups of the liquid each day. This broth rehydrates the body, replaces lost minerals, and will help you feel better faster.

Sound Therapy

Music and relaxation, a music therapy program in which clients practice stress-reduction techniques to music until the sound itself triggers the relaxation response, can help relieve diarrhea linked to stress or tension.

Sound-healing approaches include projecting sound into the body and toning; the sound vibrations created during these treatments are said to positively affect the body's internal energy balance.

Prevention

When traveling to developing countries, be careful about what you eat and drink. Don't eat foods that are raw or unpeeled, and don't drink water from a tap, well, or stream unless you know it's been sterilized. Better to play it safe and drink only bottled beverages—served without ice. Remember that harmful bacteria trapped in ice will be released into your glass when the ice melts. Keep the following homeopathic remedies in your travel bag in case you do get a case of Montezuma's revenge:

- *Arsenicum album* (12x) for burning diarrhea.
- *Nux vomica* (12x) for painful, cramping diarrhea from bad food or water.
- *Phosphorus* (12x) for painless diarrhea that is exhausting. ∎

*E*arache

Symptoms

- Pain in the ear that is either sharp and sudden or dull and throbbing, accompanied by fever, nasal congestion, and muffled hearing, may indicate otitis media (middle ear infection). A child with otitis media may tug at the ear and cry when lying down at night.

- Itching in the ear, later with sharp or dull pain that worsens when you pull on the earlobe, may indicate swimmer's ear. There may also be a yellowish discharge, and possibly fever and temporary hearing loss.

- Sudden ear pain, usually after an injury or infection, may indicate a ruptured eardrum. There may also be bleeding or pus discharge from the ear, dizziness, ringing in the ear, or partial hearing loss.

Call Your Doctor If

- body temperature rises above 101°F or 102°F; a fever signals the possibility of a more serious infection requiring medical attention.

- you or your child frequently develops otitis media; repeated bouts with the disorder can lead to hearing loss or more serious infections.

- you suspect that you or your child has hearing problems; an infection may be affecting the ability to hear.

- you suspect that your young child has otitis media.

- you suspect you have a ruptured eardrum; you may need antibiotics or in some cases surgery.

P ain in the ear can indicate any of a number of conditions, from excessive earwax to temporomandibular joint syndrome. But it is most often the result of otitis media, or infection of the middle ear. Earache is also often caused by swimmer's ear—inflammation and possibly infection of the outer ear canal.

Treatment Options

Most treatments try to rid the ear of infection or provide relief while the infection clears up on its own. Controversy surrounds the use of antibiotics. For example, research indicates that 80 percent of otitis media cases are viral in origin and therefore will not respond to antibiotics. But many doctors, particularly in the U.S., are concerned that without antibiotics, bacteria lurking inside the middle ear can grow out of control, possibly causing a serious complication such as hearing loss or mastoiditis. To be on the safe side, many American physicians treat all otitis media cases as if bacteria were present.

■ Aromatherapy
Lavender *(Lavandula angustifolia)* oil may help reduce inflammation and pain. For swimmer's ear, gently rub the area around the outer ear with 3 to 5 drops of lavender oil diluted in 1 tsp vegetable oil.

■ Ayurvedic Medicine
To open and drain the Eustachian tubes, Ayurvedic physicians massage the lymph nodes outside the ears. The massage is complemented with a drink made with the herb amala, a source of vitamin C.

■ Herbal Therapy
Mullein *(Verbascum thapsus)* oil, which has anti-inflammatory properties, may help soothe and heal an inflamed ear canal. Put 1 to 3 drops in the infected ear every three hours. Because ear-drop solutions cannot penetrate the middle ear, they should be reserved for outer ear infections. CAUTION: Do not use ear drops if there's a chance that the eardrum is ruptured.

■ Homeopathy
In the early stages of an ear infection with sudden onset and feverish restlessness, use *Aconite* (30c).

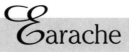

arache

For children with otitis media who are very irritable and in great pain, try *Chamomilla* (30c). When a child is weepy, clingy, feels better in the open air, and has a yellowish green discharge from the nose, use *Pulsatilla* (30c) every four to six hours. If the pain is severe, take 30c every half-hour until the pain abates, then take it every four to six hours.

▩ Nutrition and Diet
The following supplements will help fight a viral infection:
- Vitamin C. Daily dosage: Your child's age times 500 mg. (WARNING: High doses of vitamin C can cause diarrhea; spread the dose out evenly during the day. Many people cannot tolerate more than 1,000 mg every two hours.)
- Zinc. Daily dosage: Your age times 2.5 mg. Do not take more than 50 mg per day without consulting a nutritionist.
- Bioflavonoids. Daily dosage: Your child's age times 50 mg, with 250 mg as the maximum.

▩ Osteopathy
Consult an osteopathic practitioner for therapies, such as craniosacral manipulative therapy, that may help drainage of the Eustachian tubes.

Home Remedies

- Warmth, perhaps provided by a hot compress, relieves the symptoms of ear infection. Hot footbaths and inhalations of steam may also help.
- Gargling with salt water helps soothe an irritated throat and clear the Eustachian tubes.
- For swimmer's ear, make sure you keep the infected ear canal dry during the healing process, even while showering. Use earplugs or a shower cap.
- Some people find relief with over-the-counter nasal sprays, which act as decongestants. Used for more than three days, however, sprays can become habit forming and lead to rebound congestion, or a worsening of your condition.

Prevention

Because bottle-fed babies are more likely to get otitis media, it is better to breast-feed your infant, if possible, to prevent ear infections. (If you must bottle-feed, never lay your baby down and prop the bottle up.) Also, because allergies can cause otitis media, remove as many environmental pollutants from your home as you can, including dust, cleaning fluid and solvents, and tobacco smoke.

Food allergies may play a role in otitis media, so if you or your child is susceptible to the disease, try cutting back on milk, wheat products, corn products, and food additives, as these tend to be more allergenic than other foods. ■

Middle Ear Infection

Excess fluid in the middle ear normally drains harmlessly into the throat via the Eustachian tube. But if this tiny conduit becomes infected—perhaps by the same organisms that bring on a cold or the flu—it can swell shut, trapping fluid in the middle ear and promoting further infection. This fluid buildup causes painful pressure that, without proper treatment, can eventually burst the eardrum.

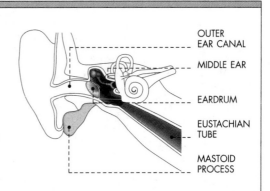

Fever and Chills

Symptoms

- A higher-than-normal body temperature (usually above 98.6°F), with or without other symptoms; possibly chills, especially while the fever is climbing.

- Fever (102°F to 106°F) that comes on abruptly, possibly accompanied by chills, headache, malaise, diarrhea, runny nose, dry cough, sore throat, or aches in muscles or joints. You may have the flu or some other viral infection.

- Fever after several hours in the heat; you could have heat exhaustion.

Call Your Doctor If

- you have fever with a severe headache and a stiff neck, possibly accompanied by nausea, vomiting, sensitivity to light, drowsiness, or confusion. These are signs of meningitis.

- a baby or child has fever with convulsions, shaking, and/or a blue color to the face. Call 911 or your emergency number immediately.

- a child under age 12 has fever along with earache, rash, swollen jaw, noisy breathing, runny nose, red eyes, or dry cough. The problem could be an ear infection, croup, measles, German measles, chickenpox, or mumps.

- you have fever accompanied by throbbing face pain, especially when a tooth is touched. You probably have a tooth abscess; call your dentist now for emergency treatment. *(See Toothache, pages 132-133.)*

I t may be difficult to appreciate the benefits when your body feels like it's on fire, but fever is a remarkable and extremely valuable defense mechanism. Fever itself is not an illness; it's a symptom of one. An elevated temperature is one of the first indications that foreign invaders have entered your body and that your immune system is responding to the threat. Perhaps more important is the direct role fever plays in battling these intruders. By turning up the heat, the body actually slows the growth of disease-causing bacteria and viruses, rendering them more vulnerable to defender cells of the immune system.

A fever is often preceded by chills or a sensation of overwhelming coldness. Although the two would seem to have contrasting effects, fever and chills are actually part of the same process. When the body comes under attack, blood vessels constrict and retreat inward to prevent heat loss. The skin begins to feel colder, prompting the body to fire up its heat-generating mechanism—shivering. This rapid, involuntary muscle movement quickly warms you up.

Although fever is usually the result of an infection, it can also be brought on by a number of other conditions. Fever is often a symptom of dehydration or anxiety, for example, and it can accompany such serious disorders as nerve disease and cancer. But just because you have a fever doesn't always mean there's something wrong with you. In healthy people, vigorous exercise can raise the body temperature well above normal.

Treatment Options

Acupressure
Applying pressure to a number of points is often recommended for fever, chills, and other symptoms that may accompany the flu; Spleen 6 and Stomach 36 are recommended for stimulating natural resistance to colds and flu *(see page 67 for the locations of these points)*. Large Intestine 11 *(opposite)* may help fight fever and strengthen your immune system.

Ayurvedic Medicine
An Ayurvedic physician may recommend one of the following remedies, depending on the exact nature of your constitution: for general fever and chills, a powder or milk decoction of the root of

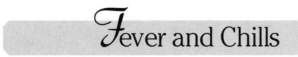 Fever and Chills

shatavari or an infusion or powder of Indian basil; for fever and colds without chills, an infusion or powder of mint; for general fever, solidified starch from a decoction of *guduchi.*

Flower Remedy
The Bach Rescue Remedy is often recommended for fever. Consult a naturopath or other practitioner familiar with flower remedies.

Herbal Therapies
For an herbal approach to stimulating your immune system, try taking ½ tsp each of tincture of goldenseal *(Hydrastis canadensis)* and echinacea *(Echinacea* spp.) twice a day. An infusion of boneset *(Eupatorium perfoliatum)* may relieve aches and fever: Simmer 1 cup boiling water with 2 tsp of the herb for 10 to 15 minutes; drink a cupful every hour, as hot as you can stand it. To combat chills, try taking 30 drops of yarrow *(Achillea millefolium)* or elder *(Sambucus nigra)* flower tincture every four hours until your chills are gone.

Homeopathy
Homeopathic remedies are particularly good for fevers; homeopathic physicians find them more effective than conventional medications such as aspirin, acetaminophen, or ibuprofen. A practitioner might recommend the following: for a mild or moderate fever, *Ferrum phosphoricum*; for acute fever, *Aconite* or *Belladonna*; for fever with extreme chills, *Bryonia.*

Hydrotherapy
Most hydrotherapists would not try to reduce a slight fever (between 99°F and 102°F) and in some cases might even attempt to encourage or increase the fever to enhance its germ-fighting abilities. Consult a healthcare practitioner familiar with hydrotherapy techniques.

To lower a fever, a hydrotherapist might recommend a wet sheet pack: Place two blankets on a bed, leaving a substantial portion of each blanket hanging over the sides. Spread a wet, wrung-out cotton sheet on the bed and have the patient lie on it. Wrap the sheet first around the trunk and legs, then the arms; fold the sheet under at the feet to cover them completely. Next, cover the patient with a blanket, using a towel at the neck and shoulders to prevent draft. The sheet pack should remain in place for 12 to 20 minutes. Repeat the application once if necessary.

Nutrition and Diet
Fever can leave you exhausted, so it's important to rebuild your body's defenses through a nutritious diet once the storm has passed. When your temperature returns to normal, be sure to eat plenty of vegetables, fruits, proteins, and whole-grain cereals.

Home Remedies

- Avoid dehydration by drinking plenty of fluids, including water, tea, fruit juice, and broth.
- Suck on cubes of ice or frozen fruit juice.
- Take a warm bath; water that is too cool can make you shiver, possibly raising your body temperature even more. Sponging off with water can also help, but be careful not to get chilled.
- Eat if you feel hungry, but don't force it. The old myth about starving a fever is just that— a myth. ■

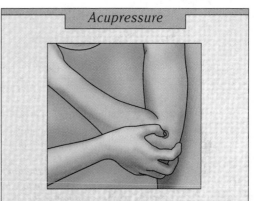

Acupressure

Large Intestine 11 • *Use this point to combat fever and strengthen your immune system. With your arm bent, use your thumb to press deeply on the outer edge of the elbow crease. Repeat on the other arm.*

$\mathcal{F}$lu

Symptoms

- Fever—usually between 101°F and 102°F, but occasionally as high as 106°F—sometimes alternating with chills.

- Sore throat.

- Dry, hacking cough.

- Aching muscles.

- General fatigue and weakness.

- Nasal congestion, sneezing.

- Headache.

Call Your Doctor If

- you experience any of these symptoms and your immune system is already weakened by cancer, diabetes, AIDS, or other conditions; or if you have a serious illness like chronic heart or kidney disease, impaired breathing, cystic fibrosis, or chronic anemia. You may be at risk for developing serious secondary complications and need to be carefully monitored as long as symptoms last.

- your fever lasts more than three or four days, you become short of breath while resting, or you have chest pain. You may have developed pneumonia.

I nfluenza—commonly shortened to "flu"—is an extremely contagious viral disease that appears most frequently in winter and early spring. The infection spreads through your upper respiratory tract and sometimes goes into your lungs. The virus typically sweeps through large groups of people who share indoor space, such as schools, offices, and nursing homes.

Although both colds and influenza stem from viruses that infect the upper respiratory tract, the symptoms of influenza are more pronounced and its complications more severe. Influenza occurs most commonly in school-age children, but its most severe effects are felt by infants, the elderly, and people with chronic ailments. Specific strains of the disease can be prevented by injections of antibodies in a flu vaccine, but after influenza—or any other viral infection—has started, there is no cure except to let it run its course.

Treatment Options

Alternative therapies may help strengthen your body's ability to fight the virus and can help ease temporary flu symptoms.

Aromatherapy

In flu season, when those around you are coming down with the virus, protect yourself by gargling daily with 1 drop each of the essential oils of tea tree *(Melaleuca alternifolia)* and lemon in a glass of

Acupressure

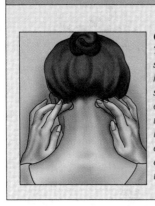

Gall Bladder 20
To help relieve flu symptoms, including headaches and eyestrain, place the tips of your middle fingers in the hollows at the base of your skull, about two inches apart on either side of the spine. Press firmly.

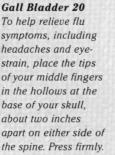
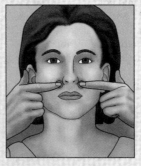

Large Intestine 20
This point can help relieve nasal congestion associated with the flu. Using your index or middle fingers, press hard on the outer edge of the nostrils at the base of the nose.

Flu

warm water; stir well before each mouthful. Do not swallow. If you come down with the flu despite your best preventive efforts, 10 to 20 drops of tea tree in a hot bath may help your immune system fight the viral infection and ease your symptoms. Be sure to use a pure, unadulterated form of tea tree oil; adulterated forms can be irritating to the skin.

If you have a congested nose or chest, add a few drops of essential oils of eucalyptus globulus *(E. globulus)* or peppermint *(Mentha piperita)* to a steam vaporizer. If you are asthmatic, be cautious the first time you try this; if you have not been exposed to essential oils before, inhaling the vapor may actually precipitate an attack.

■ Herbal Therapies

For an herbal approach to stimulating your immune system, try taking ½ tsp each of tincture of goldenseal *(Hydrastis canadensis)* and echinacea *(Echinacea* spp.) twice a day. If flu symptoms appear, chew a clove of raw garlic *(Allium sativum)* for its antiviral properties, but do not eat raw garlic on an empty stomach.

An infusion of boneset *(Eupatorium perfoliatum)* may relieve aches and fever and clear congestion: Simmer 1 cup boiling water with 2 tsp of the herb for 10 to 15 minutes; drink a cupful every hour, as hot as you can stand it. To combat chills, try taking 30 drops of yarrow *(Achillea millefolium)* or elder *(Sambucus nigra)* flower tincture every four hours until your chills are gone.

■ Homeopathy

For homeopathic self-care, try one of the following remedies in 6c or 30c dosages every six to eight hours for a day or two. If you don't notice an improvement in your condition after 24 hours, try another homeopathic remedy.

- If you feel tired, weak, and chilled, with a dull headache and stuffy nose, try *Gelsemium.*
- If you feel general achiness with irritability and have a headache that is worse when you move around, and if you are thirsty for cold fluids and have a dry hacking cough, try *Bryonia.*
- If you are restless, chilled, and thirsty, with a dry mouth, hoarse voice, and aching joints, try *Rhus toxicodendron.*

■ Nutrition and Diet

Eat vitamin C-rich fresh fruits and vegetables like citrus fruits, Brussels sprouts, and strawberries, or take 1,000 mg of vitamin C every two to three hours when awake. Increase zinc intake with lean meats, fish, and whole-grain breads and cereals.

■ Reflexology

To support your respiratory system, press your thumb into the solar plexus/diaphragm area on your foot for a few seconds, or massage the area with your thumb.

Home Remedies

- If you have a sore or scratchy throat, try a salt-water gargle. Dissolve 1 tsp salt in 1 pt warm water. Gargle whenever your throat is uncomfortable, but don't swallow the mixture.
- Use a heating pad on body aches.
- When you feel like eating, try bland, starchy foods like dry toast, bananas, applesauce, cottage cheese, boiled rice, rice pudding, cooked cereal, and baked potatoes. These foods provide a gentle transition for your digestive system when you have not been eating regularly.
- Don't drink alcoholic beverages; they leave you dehydrated and can lower your body's ability to fight illness and secondary infection.

Prevention

The most effective preventive measure against influenza is to be inoculated every fall against strains that have developed since the previous outbreak. If you are vaccinated against one or more type A and B strains, you may still come down with flu, but your symptoms are likely to be milder than they would have been had you not had a vaccination.

- Give up smoking and alcohol; both lower your resistance to infection.
- Avoid sleeping in a room with someone who has the flu; the virus is easily spread in the air.
- Wash your hands often to kill viruses you may have picked up by touching contaminated objects like doorknobs or phone receivers. ■

Food Poisoning

Symptoms

Generally, food poisoning causes some combination of nausea, vomiting, and diarrhea that may or may not be bloody, sometimes with other symptoms.

- Abdominal cramps, diarrhea, and vomiting, starting from one hour to four days after eating tainted food and lasting up to four days, usually indicate bacterial food poisoning.

- Vomiting, diarrhea, abdominal cramps, headaches, and fever and chills, beginning from 12 to 48 hours after eating contaminated food—particularly seafood —usually indicate viral food poisoning.

- Vomiting, diarrhea, sweating, dizziness, tearing in the eyes, excessive salivation, mental confusion, and stomach pain, beginning about 30 minutes after eating contaminated food, are typical indications of chemical food poisoning.

- Partial loss of speech or vision, muscle paralysis from the head down through the body, and vomiting may indicate botulism, a severe but very rare type of bacterial food poisoning.

Call Your Doctor If

- you recognize symptoms of botulism. You need immediate medical treatment for a life-threatening illness.

- you recognize symptoms of chemical food poisoning. You need immediate medical treatment to avoid potential damage to one or more of your vital organs.

- the vomiting or diarrhea is severe and lasts for more than two days. You are at risk of becoming dehydrated, which can be dangerous.

Y ou can get food poisoning after eating food contaminated by viral, bacterial, or chemical agents. Food poisoning causes mild to acute discomfort and may leave you temporarily dehydrated. Mild cases last only a few hours or at worst a day or two, but some types—such as botulism or certain forms of chemical poisoning—are severe and possibly life threatening unless you get medical treatment.

Types of Food Poisoning

Many bacteria can cause food poisoning. People who have a staph infection or are infected with staph bacteria can transmit them to food they are preparing. People who eat or drink contaminated food or water can get traveler's diarrhea, usually caused by the bacterium E. coli. Bacteria can contaminate poultry, eggs, and meat, causing salmonella poisoning; though potentially fatal, most cases cause only mild discomfort. Harmful bacteria grow in cooked and raw meat and fish, dairy products, and prepared foods left at room temperature too long; dishes made with mayonnaise are notorious culprits.

Canned goods—especially home-canned produce—can harbor an anaerobic bacterium that is not destroyed by cooking. This bacterium causes botulism, a rare but potentially fatal food poisoning. Infants may develop botulism from eating honey because their immature digestive systems cannot neutralize its naturally occurring bacteria.

Raw seafood—especially contaminated shellfish—may bring on viral food poisoning. Certain mushrooms, berries, and other plants are naturally poisonous to humans and should never be eaten; potato sprouts and eyes also contain natural toxins. Toxic mold can form on improperly stored fruit, vegetables, grains, and nuts. Chemical food poisoning can be caused by pesticides or by keeping food in unsanitary containers.

Treatment Options

Vomiting and diarrhea are the body's way of flushing poison out of your system, so don't take any antiemetic or antidiarrheal medicine for 24 hours after your symptoms develop. Once you can keep fluid in your stomach, drink clear liquids for about

*F*ood Poisoning

12 hours. Then eat bland foods like white rice, cooked cereals, and clear soups for a full day.

Because repeated vomiting or diarrhea can remove large amounts of water from your system, dehydration is a potentially dangerous complication, especially in children and older adults. You must see that lost fluids are replaced promptly and completely. If you cannot keep liquids down, intravenous fluid replacement may be necessary.

Acupressure

See the illustration below, right, for an effective acupressure technique to relieve the nausea associated with food poisoning.

Chinese Medicine

Among practitioners of Chinese medicine, *Po Chai* and Pill Curing are well-known herbal formulas for treating food poisoning.

Flower Remedy

The remedy Crab Apple is often recommended for food poisoning. Consult a naturopath or other practitioner familiar with flower remedies.

Herbal Therapies

For nausea, try ginger *(Zingiber officinale):* Take two capsules or a cup of ginger tea every two hours as needed. An infusion of meadowsweet *(Filipendula ulmaria),* catnip *(Nepeta cataria),* or slippery elm *(Ulmus fulva)* may help soothe the stomach: Steep 2 tsp of the herb in a cup of boiling water for 15 minutes; drink three times daily.

Homeopathy

Try any of the following over-the-counter remedies in 12c potency every three to four hours until symptoms improve: *Arsenicum album, Veratrum album, Nux vomica,* or *Podophyllum.*

Hydrotherapy

For symptom relief, alternate hot and cold compresses on your abdomen, with five minutes of hot followed by 10 minutes of cold. Hydrotherapists also recommend taking medicinal charcoal internally. Take two to three capsules after each bout of diarrhea; dissolve the tablets in water and drink.

Nutrition and Diet

After symptoms subside, restore strength by eating foods like white rice, bland vegetables, mashed potatoes, and bananas. To restore essential bacteria to your digestive tract, eat plain yogurt with active *Lactobacillus acidophilus* cultures, or take *Lactobacillus acidophilus* capsules. Avoid unfermented milk products, which may be difficult to digest.

Prevention

- Always wash your hands before preparing any food; wash utensils with hot soapy water after using them to prepare any meat or fish.
- Don't thaw frozen meat at room temperature. Thaw it gradually in a refrigerator, or thaw it quickly in a microwave oven and cook at once.
- Avoid uncooked marinated food and raw meat, fish, or eggs; cook all such food thoroughly.
- Don't eat any food that looks or smells spoiled, or any food from bulging cans or cracked jars.
- Set your refrigerator at 37°F; never eat cooked meat or dairy products that have been out of a refrigerator more than two hours.
- To relieve general nausea, try pressing Pericardium 6—on your inner forearm, two finger widths from the wrist *(below).* ∎

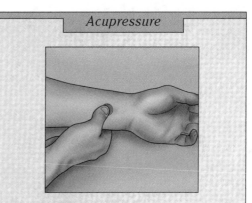

Acupressure

Pericardium 6 • *To relieve general nausea, try pressing this point—on your inner forearm, two finger widths from the wrist crease—for one minute. Repeat on the other arm.*

Gas and Gas Pains

Symptoms

- Abdominal bloating and pain.
- Belching.
- Flatulence (passing rectal gas).

Call Your Doctor If

- you have persistent, unexplained bloating for more than three days; you may have a more severe abdominal disorder.
- you have severe abdominal pain; you may have appendicitis.
- you have pain in your upper right abdomen; you might have gallstones or a stomach ulcer.
- you are flatulent, are losing weight, and have pale, foul-smelling bowel movements; you might have a malabsorption disorder, in which your intestines are not able to digest fat.

Gas and gas pains are a normal part of your digestive process. People may typically pass gas more than 10 times a day, but you can greatly exceed that average and still be perfectly healthy. You can usually prevent and treat gas and gas pains without professional care, but if you have other symptoms, you should consult a doctor to find out if you have a more serious health problem.

Treatment Options

Changes in diet—avoiding or limiting milk products, alcohol, carbonated beverages, and high-fiber foods like beans—can go a long way toward solving problems with excessive gas. Many people rely on over-the-counter medications containing the active ingredient simethicone, which can help break up gas bubbles in the large intestine. Alternative medicine offers a wide variety of natural treatments as well.

Acupressure
Pressing the following points may help to alleviate gas pains: Conception Vessel 6, Large Intestine 4, Spleen 6, and Stomach 36. (See the illustration opposite and on pages 65 and 67 for information on point locations.)

Acupuncture
A practitioner can provide treatment for gas using the same points used in acupressure.

Exercise
Moderate exercise after meals can help move gas through your system more quickly. In addition, following a regular program of exercise stimulates digestion and promotes the reabsorption and expulsion of gas.

Herbal Therapies
Anise water, made by steeping 1 tsp aniseeds in 1 cup water for 10 minutes, may be helpful. Teas made with peppermint (Mentha piperita), chamomile (Matricaria recutita), or fennel (Foeniculum vulgare) may also relieve gas pains.

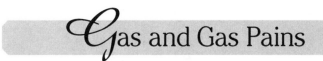 Gas and Gas Pains

▮ Homeopathy

Carbo vegetabilis is the most commonly used homeopathic remedy, but *Lycopodium* is used as well. *Nux vomica* is used for gas associated with constipation, and *Chamomilla* is preferred for gas in infants. Talk to a homeopath about which is most suitable for you.

▮ Hydrotherapy

To relieve gas pains, apply a hot compress (a washcloth soaked in hot water and then wrung out) to the abdomen for several minutes, then follow with a cold friction rub: Soak a washcloth in ice water, wring it out, and rub it briskly over the abdomen for about half a minute.

▮ Nutrition and Diet

Increase your fiber intake slowly and try avoiding beans, peas, and fermented foods such as cheese, soy sauce, and alcohol. Asafetida powder dispels intestinal gas and may be used as a spice with beans. Drink fewer carbonated drinks. Avoid mixing proteins and carbohydrates at the same meal. Do not overeat, and eat fewer different food items at one sitting. For people who are lactose intolerant, replacing cow's milk with soybean milk or using lactose-reduced dairy products may help.

▮ Reflexology

Consult a certified reflexologist for area locations that can be manipulated to help the digestive process in the stomach and intestines.

▮ Yoga

Any of the yoga postures that compress and stretch the abdomen help stimulate digestion and thus reduce gas and bloating. Try the Bow *(see page 107)*, Cobra *(see page 38)*, or Pigeon positions *(see page 14)*.

Home Remedies

Dissolve a teaspoon or two of superfine white, green, or yellow French clay (available at health food stores) in water and drink at least once daily (but not with meals). The clay absorbs impurities and intestinal gas; check with your doctor to make sure it won't absorb medications you may be taking.

Prevention

One of the main methods of preventing gas and gas pains is also the primary treatment: Avoid foods that generate gas in your system. Try to become more aware of the air that you swallow. You can avoid some gas, for instance, by not gulping your food; chew your food slowly and thoroughly. ▮

Acupressure

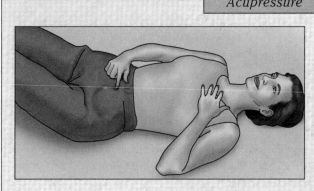

Conception Vessel 6 • *Pressing on Conception Vessel 6 may help relieve gas pains. Measure three finger widths below the navel, then press inward on this point as far as you can, using your index finger. Inhale slowly and deeply, relaxing as you exhale.*

out

Symptoms

- Sudden, intense pain in a joint, typically the big toe or ankle, sometimes the knee.
- Swelling, inflammation, and a feeling that the joint is very hot.
- In extreme cases, alternating chills and fever.
- Usually strikes unexpectedly and may recur, but the symptoms typically do not last more than a week.

Call Your Doctor If

- severe pain in a joint recurs or lasts more than a few days, especially if the pain is accompanied by chills or fever; you may be experiencing the early signs of rheumatoid arthritis.

ithout warning and, for some reason, in the middle of the night, it strikes—an intense pain in a joint, most often the big toe. With prompt treatment, the pain and inflammation of gout disappear after a few days, but they may recur at any time. Nine out of 10 sufferers are middle-aged men, and about half of them have a hereditary predisposition to the ailment.

Gout is uncommon in women and very rare in children. Men who are overweight or are suffering from high blood pressure are particularly prone to gout, which is actually a form of arthritis brought on by an excessively high level of uric acid in the blood. Specifically, it is the body's reaction to irritating crystalline deposits in the space between the bones in a joint.

Treatment Options

Nonconventional approaches to treating gout begin with reducing the immediate pain and inflammation, then continue with controlling excessive uric acid production. If you suspect that you have gout, you should consult a physician; left untreated, uric acid deposits can eventually cause irreversible damage to the kidneys and other tissues.

Acupuncture

Because acupuncture can be administered to areas other than the swollen joint, this procedure may be better tolerated than direct treatments, such as massage, by patients in the initial stages of gout. See a professional for treatment, which will focus on providing relief from the symptoms of acute pain and inflammation.

Herbal Therapies

Drink an infusion of 2 tsp celery *(Apium graveolens)* seed or gravelroot *(Eupatorium purpureum)* in a cup of water, three times a day, to stimulate elimination of uric acid. Do not take herbal teas if colchicine has been prescribed.

Homeopathy

A homeopathic physician may consider predisposition to gout in an overall constitutional treatment. *Colchicum,* or autumn crocus, from which colchicine is extracted, can be effective in relieving the pain of an attack. *Bryonia* may help when there is

Acupressure

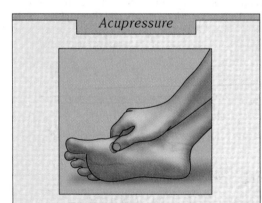

Spleen 3 • *To relieve the pain of a gouty toe, locate the indentation on the inside of the affected foot, just behind the bulge made by the large joint of the big toe. Maintain pressure on the point site with your thumb for 60 seconds. Repeat on the other foot.*

G

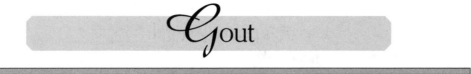

Joint Problems

*Gout occurs when the body is unable
to rid the blood of excess uric acid.
Crystals of the chemical accumulate
between the bones of certain joints,
most commonly in the big toe. The
result can be sudden and severe pain,
inflammation, and in severe cases,
joint deformity.*

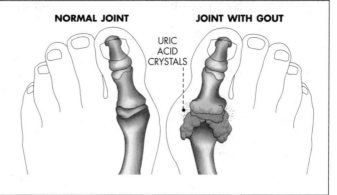

NORMAL JOINT   JOINT WITH GOUT

URIC
ACID
CRYSTALS

severe pain from slight movement of the affected
joint. Other mixed homeopathic remedies may include dilute doses of *Arnica, Ledum, Urtica urens,
Benzoicum acidum, Lycopodium*, and *Pulsatilla*.

Nutrition and Diet
In general, gout seems more common in people
with diets that include meat and animal fats and is
unusual in those following vegetarian diets. Dietary
regimens for preventing attacks of gout in people
showing a hereditary predisposition to the disease
usually eliminate red meat and meat extracts such
as bouillon and gravies; yeast and other enzyme-
producing products; organ meats such as liver,
sweetbreads, and kidneys; shellfish and certain
kinds of preserved fish, including sardines, herring,
and anchovies.

Vitamin C (1,000 mg three times a day) may
help with the excretion of uric acid; consult a
physician or healthcare practitioner familiar
with nutritional therapies when taking large doses
of vitamin C, which can cause some side effects.
Some naturopathic practitioners also recommend
supplementing the diet with 1 to 2 tbsp of flaxseed
oil a day.

Several authorities report favorable results in
treating the pain of chronic gout by having patients
eat fresh or canned cherries—up to 8 oz a day—
or drink cherry juice. Similar effects are claimed
for strawberries, blueberries, and other red-blue
berries.

Drinking plenty of clear, nonalcoholic fluids—
fruit juices, herbal teas, or water—helps to dilute
the urine and promote excretion of uric acid
through continued flushing of the kidneys.

Reflexology
To help restore balance to the kidneys, the organs
responsible for uric acid production, a reflexology
practitioner will work the appropriate areas related
to the kidneys; this should be done on both feet.
In addition to affecting the kidneys, this technique
may also serve to break up deposits of uric acid
crystals that have become concentrated in the feet.

Home Remedies

The first concern in an attack of gout is to reduce
pain and inflammation. If you can stand it, apply a
plastic bag containing a few ice cubes or a bag of
frozen vegetables to the joint; this will help relieve
painful swelling. Wrap the cold bag in a soft cloth
or towel and hold it against the painful area for up
to five minutes at a time, then repeat as needed.

Prevention

If gouty arthritis runs in the family, men in particular should moderate their intake of alcohol, fats,
and foods high in purines (chemicals essential to
the production of uric acid), and they should keep
their weight within recommended ranges. ∎

G

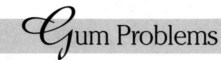

Gum Problems

Symptoms

- Swollen, red gums that may bleed easily.

- Localized pain, loose teeth, and bad breath, which suggest periodontitis, an inflammation of the periodontal ligament; x-rays may reveal some bone loss in the jaw area.

- Extremely painful, inflamed gums coated with a grayish white mucus; sometimes accompanied by a mild fever, malaise, bad breath, excess saliva, and painful swallowing. These are signs of Vincent's angina, also known as trench mouth.

- Sudden and unexplained severe bone loss around molars and incisors, especially in young African American girls; this is indicative of juvenile periodontitis.

- Extremely sore, swollen gums that bleed easily; perhaps accompanied by earaches, a sinuslike infection, nosebleeds, fever, weight loss, and malaise. You may have Wegener's granulomatosis, a rare but potentially fatal disease.

Call Your Dentist If

- you have any of the groups of symptoms listed above; timely treatment can help prevent the spread of infection and potentially save teeth.

P *eriodontal disease (gum disease)—an infection of the gums and other tissues that support the teeth—is one of the most prevalent of all chronic diseases. A diet rich in refined sugars is largely to blame, but modern dentistry and good toothbrushes and toothpastes have helped offset some of the pernicious effects of our eating habits; as a result, only 8 percent of adults ever develop severe gum problems. That rate would be even lower if people made an effort to cut back on highly processed foods, notorious for their refined-sugar content, and took dental hygiene more seriously.*

Treatment Options

The best treatment for periodontal disease is prevention. If you do develop gum problems, seek professional treatment and advice. Many alternative therapies exist for gum problems, including rinses and pastes that will reduce plaque, fight infection and inflammation, and slow bleeding. But these remedies are no better than conventional commercial products at reaching below the gum line to areas where periodontitis blossoms. You still need to see a dentist regularly to ward off the risk of severe gum disease and tooth loss.

Acupuncture
A licensed acupuncture practitioner may choose areas that would stimulate the immune system to help fight off infections in the gums and reduce inflammation and pain.

Herbal Therapies
Massage gums with an infusion of goldenseal *(Hydrastis canadensis)* or myrrh *(Commiphora molmol)* to fight infection. Gargle with bayberry *(Myrica* spp.) or prickly ash *(Zanthoxylum americanum)* to stimulate circulation. A combination of sage *(Salvia officinalis)* and chamomile *(Matricaria recutita)* in an infusion makes an excellent mouthwash. You might also try gargling with echinacea *(Echinacea* spp.) tea made with 1 ml echinacea tincture in a small glass of water. Make a tea by boiling 1 to 2 tsp of the root in 1 cup of water; simmer for 10 minutes. Or drink Roman chamomile *(Anthemis nobilis)* or myrrh tea to fight inflammation in the gums. CAUTION: Do not use myrrh if you are pregnant.

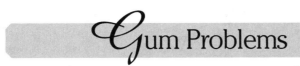Gum Problems

Homeopathy

For tender, bleeding gums and excessive salivation try *Mercurius vivus*; take orally twice a day for three days. If you continue to have problems, see a professional homeopath.

Massage

Massaging the gums can improve circulation and speed healing. Use the rounded part of your fingertips and move along your gum line inside your mouth, or from the outside press on the gums through your cheek. A stimulator brush, which has only two rows of bristles and is used without toothpaste, can also be therapeutic.

Nutrition and Diet

Crucial for healthy gums is a diet low in refined sugars and high in fiber. Other important nutritional elements include vitamins A (especially beta carotene), C, and E, as well as zinc, flavonoids (present in onions), and folic acid (particularly for pregnant women and women on oral contraceptives). Gingivitis, the earliest stage of periodontal disease, is common in scurvy patients, a reflection of vitamin C's vital role in maintaining a healthy mouth.

Home Remedies

You can make a wide assortment of mouthwashes and toothpastes at home. Some of the most effective ingredients include:

- a combination of baking soda and hydrogen peroxide, for brushing your teeth or as a mouth rinse.
- a mixture of bayberry and prickly ash as a gargle.
- cashew oil, vitamin E oil, or poultices of goldenseal or myrrh massaged into the gums, to speed healing and protect against infection.

Prevention

For proper dental care you need to floss daily, brush longer, rinse with a mouthwash, and massage your gum line. Always floss first, to loosen food particles and plaque, then brush your teeth gently but thoroughly with a soft brush using a circular motion. Rigorous horizontal brushing with hard bristles can cause your gums to recede. Mouthwashes combat bacteria, but they should not be substituted for brushing, which you should do two or three times a day.

The American Dental Association (ADA) recommends that you visit your dentist once or twice a year to get rid of intractable plaque and calculus, but some dentists believe that excellent at-home dental hygiene keeps the plaque and calculus from ever forming. To achieve "excellence" you have to spend at least 15 minutes twice a day working on your teeth, and another 15 minutes a day massaging your gums. ∎

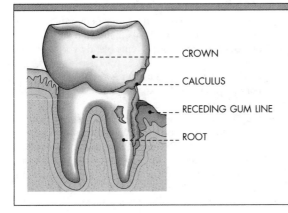

CROWN

CALCULUS

RECEDING GUM LINE

ROOT

Periodontal Disease

A bacterial film called plaque can accumulate along the gum line at the base of the teeth if not brushed away. Plaque hardens into calculus, which irritates the gums and causes them to recede. Pockets that form between the gums and teeth collect more plaque and calculus, causing destruction of the bone and ligament supporting the tooth, eventually resulting in tooth loss.

$\mathcal{H}$ay Fever

Symptoms

Attacks, often seasonal, of:

- Prolonged, sometimes violent sneezing.
- Itchy, painful nose, throat, and roof of mouth.
- Nasal discharge.
- Stuffy, runny nose.
- Postnasal drip, resulting in coughing.
- Watery, itchy eyes.
- Head and nasal congestion.
- Ear pressure or fullness.
- Lethargy; sleep disturbance or insomnia.

Call Your Doctor If

- your condition becomes so severe that it interferes with your life and you're unable to control it with alternative therapies or over-the-counter medications. Your physician may administer prescription drugs, such as nonsedating antihistamines, to help.

- a secondary infection develops in congested sinus cavities; signs are fever, pain, a yellow or green discharge, postnasal drip, and sinus or tooth tenderness.

Acupressure

Governing Vessel 24.5 • *Pressure on this point may help relieve symptoms of hay fever. Place the tip of your middle finger at the top of the bridge of your nose, between your eyebrows. Press lightly for two minutes and breathe deeply. Do three to five times, at least twice a day.*

H ay fever is an immune disorder characterized by an allergic response to pollen grains and other substances. There are two types: seasonal, which occurs only during the time of year in which certain plants pollinate, and perennial, which occurs all year round. Typically, if you suffer from hay fever in the spring, you're probably allergic to tree pollens. Grass and weed pollens may be causing your allergic reaction during the summer. In autumn ragweed may plague you, and fungus spores cause problems from late March through November.

People with perennial hay fever are usually allergic to one or more of these outdoor agents. Perennial hay fever can also be brought on by other allergy-causing substances, or allergens. These include house-dust mites, feathers, and animal dander (the tiny skin flakes animals shed along with fur), all of which may be found in pillows, down clothing and bedding, shower curtains, heavy draperies, upholstery, and thick carpeting. Another common allergen, mold, is usually found in damp areas such as bathrooms and basements.

Treatment Options

Conventional medicine has several approaches for treating hay fever, from over-the-counter antihistamines to allergy shots. A number of alternative therapies can also help with symptom control and as preventive measures.

Aromatherapy

To ease sinus irritation, combine 5 ml niaouli (*Melaleuca viridiflora*), .5 ml German chamomile (*Matricaria recutita*), and 3 drops peppermint (*Mentha piperita*) essential oil; moisten your face and then spread a drop of this blend over your skin.

Herbal Therapies

For symptom relief, take two capsules of nettle (*Urtica dioica*) every 15 minutes during an attack, then four times a day as a maintenance dose. To help reduce inflammation, try inhaling the steam from ginger (*Zingiber officinale*) tea: Mix 2 tsp chopped or grated ginger in 2 cups boiling water and let simmer for 20 minutes. Breathe in the steam for five to seven minutes. You can use the same tea reheated to repeat this treatment several times a day.

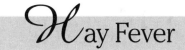ay Fever

Regular doses of parsley *(Petroselinum crispum)* may help with hay fever; it is thought to work by reducing your body's production of histamine.

You may be able to slow down your body's production of mucus with goldenrod *(Solidago virgaurea),* garlic *(Allium sativum),* or yarrow *(Achillea millefolium).* Bathe irritated eyes with compresses soaked in either eyebright *(Euphrasia officinalis)* or chamomile *(Matricaria recutita);* make a tea from the leaves and dilute it by 50 percent with water or saline solution before using it to soak the compresses.

Homeopathy

For watery, hot eyes, a burning nasal discharge with sneezing, and symptoms that feel worse late at night, try *Arsenicum album. Pulsatilla* can help if your symptoms—thick, yellow mucus accompanied by a loss of taste and smell—are made worse by warm rooms but are better outdoors. If you have watery, itchy eyes and a runny but not irritated nose, try *Euphrasia;* if, on the other hand, your nose is irritated and your eyes are watery but not itchy, try *Allium cepa.* Homeopathic practitioners recommend that you consult with a homeopath for the best treatment for conditions like hay fever because it often takes comparing as many as 15 different homeopathic remedies to find the right choice for a given individual and his or her symptoms.

Nutrition and Diet

Nutritionists believe that refined sugar and casein, the protein in dairy products, are mucus-producing substances that are best avoided during hay fever season. Taking a commercial preparation of chelated calcium and magnesium may help regulate histamine production. A diet high in fruits and vegetables will supply large amounts of vitamin C and bioflavonoids, which help stabilize the body's cells that contain histamine. Supplements of quercetin, a bioflavonoid, may also control histamine; take 250 mg four times a day, before or between meals.

Some researchers believe that honey has a desensitizing and antiallergic effect that may relieve some hay fever symptoms. Two months before the season starts, begin eating 2 tsp daily of raw honey that comes from a nearby hive. Or chew (but don't

---

OF SPECIAL INTEREST

Homemade Decongestant

Make your own decongestant by simmering grapefruit, orange, or lemon peels, including the pith, in water mixed with honey until the peels are spongy, stirring occasionally. Be careful not to overcook—you don't want candied fruit. Eat one piece when symptoms start and one piece every evening at bedtime during hay fever season. Substances in the peel and white rind act as anti-inflammatory agents and will dry mucous membranes. Lemon is considered a stimulating expectorant that may help release mucus from your lungs.

---

swallow) a bite-size piece of honeycomb for five to 10 minutes twice a day. Check with your doctor first to avoid potential allergic reactions.

Many people with hay fever are also allergic to certain foods and may experience symptoms as a result of eating such foods as eggs, nuts, fish, shellfish, chocolate, dairy products, wheat, corn, citrus fruits, or food colorings or preservatives.

Prevention

The best way to combat the allergens that are assaulting you is to avoid them. Stay indoors between six and 10 o'clock in the morning and on days when the pollen count is high. The pollen count drops on rainy days and climbs when it's hot, sunny, and windy outside.

Keep windows—in your home and car— closed and the air conditioning turned on. Change ventilation system filters in your home once a month. Remove allergens from the air with ionizing air cleaners. Prevent mold in damp basements by using space heaters and dehumidifiers.

Try to keep your grass no more than an inch high in the spring and summer so that it won't pollinate. If you do yard work, wear a filtered mask and protective glasses. Wash your face, hands, and hair and rinse your eyes when coming in from outdoors to avoid leaving traces of pollen on your pillow. ■

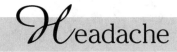eadache

Symptoms

If your headache is:

- A dull, steady pain that feels like a band tightening around your head, you have a tension headache.

- Throbbing, and it begins on one side and causes nausea, you have a migraine. Visual disturbances, such as flickering points of light, may precede the headache.

- A throbbing pain around one red, watery eye, with nasal congestion on that side of your face, you have a cluster headache.

- A steady pain behind your face that gets worse if you bend forward and is accompanied by congestion, you have a sinus headache.

Call Your Doctor If

- a severe headache is accompanied by vomiting, limb weakness, double vision, slurred speech, or difficulty in swallowing; you may have a cerebral hemorrhage or an aneurysm—get medical help now.

- your headache is of a kind you've never had, occurs first thing in the morning, is persistent, brings on vomiting, and abates during the day; you may have high blood pressure or in very rare cases a brain tumor. See your doctor without delay.

- you have a high fever, light hurts your eyes, the pain is severe and is accompanied by nausea and a stiff neck; you may have meningitis—get medical help now.

- after a head injury, you are drowsy, with dizziness, vertigo, nausea, or vomiting; you may have a concussion. See your doctor without delay.

*A*lthough painful, most headaches are minor problems treatable with aspirin or another analgesic. But if they are severe, recur often, or are attended by other symptoms, you may need to take additional steps, including consultation with your doctor.

Major Types of Headaches

Tension headaches, which afflict almost everyone at some point, bring on a dull, persistent, non-throbbing pain that can make your head feel as if it's gripped in a vise. The muscles of your neck may seem knotted, and certain areas on your head and neck may be sensitive to touch. Tension headaches can be short lived and infrequent, or enduring and chronic. They are commonly triggered by stress; but eyestrain, poor posture, too much caffeine, or the grinding of teeth at night can also cause them.

Migraines are the most debilitating of headaches; they can be completely incapacitating. A migraine usually begins with an intense, throbbing pain on one side of the head. This pain may spread and is often accompanied by nausea and vomiting. A migraine can last from a few hours to three days and can cause oversensitivity to light, odors, and sound. The various symptoms of migraines seem linked to changes in the diameter of blood vessels in the head, possibly due to an imbalance in a brain chemical known as serotonin.

Cluster headaches are so named because they tend to come in bunches. Typically they begin several hours after a person falls asleep and are sometimes preceded by a mild aching sensation on one side of the head. The pain—severe, piercing, and usually located in and around one red, watery eye —is generally accompanied by nasal congestion and a flushed face. It lasts from 30 minutes to two hours, then diminishes or disappears, only to recur perhaps a day later. The root cause is unknown.

Sinus headaches are marked by pain in the forehead, nasal area, eyes, and possibly the top of the head; they also sometimes produce a feeling of pressure behind the face. Inflammation or infection of the membranes lining the sinus cavities can give rise to such headaches, as can suction on the sinus walls, which occurs when nasal congestion creates a partial vacuum in the sinuses. Sinus headaches

$\mathcal{H}$eadache

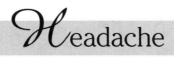

Cluster Headache

Although their exact cause is unknown, cluster headaches may arise from pressure on nerves around the eyes. Swollen sinus tissue may press against portions of these nerves, causing these electrical pathways to short-circuit and emit pain signals.

Tension Headache

Of the various types of tension headaches, one is thought to be linked to disorders in certain muscles in the head and the neck. Pain can be localized around any of these muscles or can spread to affect a broad portion of the scalp.

Sinus Headache

With a sinus headache, congestion within the sinus cavities leads to swelling that puts pressure on surrounding tissue and nerves, causing pain to radiate across the face.

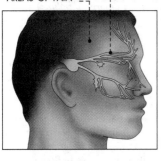

NERVES
AREAS OF PAIN

MUSCLES
AREAS OF PAIN

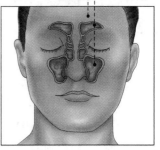

SINUS CAVITIES
AREAS OF PAIN

typically result from hay fever and other seasonal allergies, or from a cold or the flu.

Treatment Options

Alternative medicine, used alone or with conventional therapies, can be effective in dealing with headaches. Most of these remedies address the underlying causes. In particular, craniosacral therapists hope to relieve tension inside the head by manipulating the bones and membranes of the skull. Because tension so often figures in headaches, relaxation techniques are a staple of therapy.

◾ Acupressure

Follow the illustrations at the top of page 65 to locate pressure points associated with headache relief. These techniques are often used in combination with one of the aromatherapy oils at right.

◾ Aromatherapy

The following oils may ease tension or migraine headaches. Moisten your fingertips with one or two drops of lavender *(Lavandula angustifolia)* essential oil blended with a so-called carrier oil such as sunflower oil, then massage your temples with a circular motion; repeat in the hollows at the sides of your eyes, behind your ears, and over your neck. For a sinus headache, try the same techniques using Eucalyptus globulus *(E. globulus)* or wintergreen *(Gaultheria procumbens)*. For any headache, inhale a blend of lavender, rosemary *(Rosmarinus officinalis),* and peppermint *(Mentha piperita).*

◾ Chiropractic

Some tension headaches are caused by posture that puts unnecessary strain on muscles. A chiropractor may be able to remove the strain through spinal or cervical manipulation and realignment.

CONTINUED

*H*eadache

Exercise

Regular physical activity can release endorphins, the body's natural painkilling agents. Exercise may also help dilate blood vessels; this increases blood flow and may counteract the constricting action that occurs at the onset of most migraines.

To nip a tension headache in the bud, try the following exercise while breathing deeply and thinking calm thoughts: While seated, inhale and gently tip your head back until you're looking up at the ceiling (be careful not to tip your head back too far, since this can compress the cervical spine); exhale and bring your head forward until your chin rests on your chest; repeat twice.

Herbal Therapies

Perhaps the most widely recommended herbal remedy for treating and preventing migraines is feverfew *(Tanacetum parthenium),* which is

---

OF SPECIAL INTEREST

A Headache Diary

Keeping a headache diary can help you pinpoint the factors causing your specific headache patterns. The diary should provide answers to these 10 questions:

1. *When did you first develop headaches?*
2. *How often do you have them?*
3. *Do you experience symptoms prior to the headaches?*
4. *Where is the pain exactly?*
5. *How long does it last?*
6. *At what time of day do the headaches occur?*
7. *Does the eating of certain types of food precede your headaches?*
8. *If you're female, at what time in your monthly cycle do they occur?*
9. *Are the headaches triggered by physical or environmental factors, such as odor, noise, or certain kinds of weather?*
10. *What words most accurately describe the pain of your headache: throbbing, stabbing, blinding, piercing . . . ?*

---

thought to work by blocking excessive secretion of serotonin, a neurotransmitter. When blood vessels constrict in the initial stage of a migraine, serotonin is released; feverfew may help counteract this by dilating those blood vessels. Chewing a leaf or two daily is one approach to prevention, but this can occasionally cause mouth ulcers; as a substitute for the leaves, you can use 125-mg capsules. To offset an acute attack, take three or four capsules right away, then continue this dosage every four hours; don't exceed 12 capsules in a day.

Migraines brought on by stress may benefit from a combination of equal parts hawthorn *(Crataegus laevigata),* linden *(Tilia* spp.), wood betony *(Pedicularis canadensis),* skullcap *(Scutellaria lateriflora),* and cramp bark *(Viburnum opulus),* taken three times a day as a tea or tincture. For migraines accompanied by nausea, try taking 500 mg of dried ginger *(Zingiber officinale)* with water at the onset of the warning stage, if your headache pattern includes an aura; repeat every two hours if needed. Three daily doses of goldenseal *(Hydrastis canadensis)* in tincture, tea, or powdered form may help reduce sinus headache pain.

Tension headaches may respond to three daily infusions of valerian *(Valeriana officinalis)* when combined with skullcap and passionflower *(Passiflora incarnata).* Cluster headaches may get quick relief from several daily applications inside the nostrils of an over-the-counter ointment made from cayenne *(Capsicum annuum* var. *annuum).* The same ointment applied to the skin is also said to be effective in preventing migraines. Because cayenne is hot and can cause painful skin burns, it's best used under a doctor's care.

Homeopathy

A range of homeopathic medicines are available to treat specific types of headaches. For a throbbing headache that is worse on the right side when lying down, try *Belladonna.* For "splitting" headaches that feel worse with motion, noise, light, or touch, try *Bryonia.* For sinus pain with a thick nasal discharge, consider *Kali bichromicum.* For tension headaches accompanied by nausea or vomiting, try *Nux vomica.* For migraines or other chronic headaches, see a homeopathic practitioner.

$\mathcal{H}$eadache

Acupressure

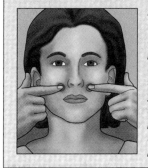

Stomach 3 • *Sinus headaches may be relieved by pressing this point. While looking in a mirror, place your index fingers at the bottom of your cheekbones, fingertips directly under the pupils of your eyes. Press firmly for one minute. Repeat three times.*

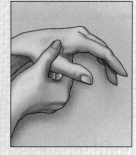

Large Intestine 4 • *Pressing this point may help relieve sinus headaches. Using the thumb and index finger of your right hand, squeeze the web of your left hand for one minute. Repeat this on the right hand. Do not use if pregnant.*

Massage

Massage therapy can relieve headache-producing tension in the muscles of your head, neck, shoulders, and face. Try giving yourself a 10-minute scalp massage: Place both middle fingers on your forehead at your hairline; using gentle pressure, gradually work them back to the crown of your head; tracing your hairline, repeat this motion in half-inch increments until you reach your temples; rotate your fingers on both sides for a few minutes; then bring both thumbs to the base of your skull along your hairline and massage both sides of your skull up to your crown to release any tightness.

Mind/Body Medicine

Meditation and progressive relaxation therapies are effective in reducing stress, which can cause tension headaches. Biofeedback training can also be helpful in controlling stress. Migraine headaches, too, can be treated through a biofeedback method called thermal biofeedback, in which you learn to increase the temperature of your hands and feet. Warming these extremities involves dilating the vessels that carry blood to them—a process that, in turn, may reduce abnormal blood vessel constriction in the skull and possibly result in diminished migraine frequency, intensity, and duration.

Nutrition and Diet

Among the foods sometimes associated with migraines are chocolate, aged cheeses, citrus fruits, processed meats containing sodium nitrates or the food additive MSG, and red wine. Keeping a food diary can help you identify foods to eliminate.

Magnesium relaxes constricted blood vessels; low levels of magnesium may contribute to migraine and cluster headaches. Supplemental doses of 200 mg three times a day may be preventive. Taking 50 to 200 mg of niacin (vitamin B_3) and niacinamide at the first hint of pain may help keep blood vessels dilated, possibly reducing the initial constriction phase of migraine headaches and thus avoiding an attack.

Osteopathy

Osteopaths believe headache pain stemming from pressure on nerves or blood vessels can be eased by neuromuscular manipulation and soft-tissue massage of your head, neck, and upper back.

Home Remedies

- Holding an ice pack or a bag of frozen vegetables against your forehead while soaking your feet in hot water may stop a migraine if done right away.
- At the first sign of a headache, drink three glasses of very cold water, then retire with a cold compress to a dark, quiet room to sleep (without a pillow).
- Inhaling pure oxygen from a tank kept near your bed may offset nighttime attacks of a cluster headache. But be sure to consult a doctor on how to use the oxygen. ∎

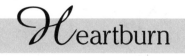 $\mathcal{H}$eartburn

Symptoms

- A burning feeling in the chest just behind the breastbone that occurs after eating and lasts a few minutes to several hours.

- Chest pain, especially after bending over or lying down.

- Burning in the throat—or hot, sour, or salty-tasting fluid at the back of the throat.

- Belching.

Call Your Doctor If

- you experience heartburn along with any of the following: difficulty swallowing, shortness of breath, sweating, dizziness, vomiting, diarrhea, extreme abdominal pain, fever, or black or bloodstained bowel movements. You may have a serious medical problem, and it could be a heart attack; call for medical help now.

- you take an antacid to relieve heartburn and do not feel relief within 15 minutes. This may also be a sign of a heart attack; call for medical help now.

- your heartburn is aggravated by exercise and relieved by rest. This can be a sign of heart disease.

- you have chronic heartburn (daily or almost daily). Your esophagus is being repeatedly burned by stomach acid, which can lead to esophagitis, esophageal scarring, stomach ulcers, or cancer.

CAUTION

Antacids can mask or aggravate some ailments. Do not take antacids without consulting your doctor if you have high blood pressure, an irregular heartbeat, kidney disease, chronic constipation, diarrhea, colitis, any kind of intestinal bleeding, or any symptoms of appendicitis. Pregnant or nursing mothers should consult a physician before taking any medication, including antacids.

Despite its name, heartburn has nothing to do with the heart. It is an irritation of the esophagus caused by stomach acid. With gravity's help, a muscular valve called the lower esophageal sphincter, or LES, keeps stomach acid in the stomach. The LES is located where the esophagus meets the stomach—below the rib cage and slightly left of center. Normally it opens to allow food into the stomach or to permit belching; then it closes again. But if the LES opens too often or too far, stomach acid can reflux, or seep, into the esophagus and cause a burning sensation.

Occasional heartburn isn't dangerous, but chronic heartburn can indicate serious problems. Heartburn is a daily occurrence for 10 percent of Americans and 50 percent of pregnant women. It's an occasional nuisance for another 30 percent of the population.

Treatment Options

Most physicians advocate antacids for occasional heartburn. A variety of antacids available over the counter work by curtailing the production of stomach acid. Alternative practitioners rely primarily on herbal remedies to reduce acid and on relaxation therapies to lessen stress.

Acupressure

To relieve heartburn, use deep thumb pressure to massage these points for at least one minute: Stomach 36, Spleen 6, and Pericardium 6. See the illustrations opposite and and on page 53 for point locations.

Chinese Medicine

Taken once or twice, a tea made from 10 grams orange peel, 4 slices fresh ginger (Zingiber officinale), 10 grams poria (Poria cocos), 10 grams agastache (Agastache rugosa), and 3 grams licorice (Glycyrrhiza glabra) may alleviate heartburn. This mixture should not be taken daily.

Herbal Therapies

Ginger (Zingiber officinale) tea can diminish heartburn quickly, and chamomile (Matricaria recutita) tea's calming effects are especially helpful for stress-related heartburn. Slippery elm (Ulmus fulva) tea is also soothing and is reputed to have

*H*eartburn

strong anti-inflammatory qualities. Mix 1 part powdered bark in 8 parts water, simmer for 10 minutes, and drink ½ cup, three times daily.

■ Homeopathy

Specific heartburn symptoms often respond well to homeopathic remedies. The dosage is 12x, taken every 15 minutes; repeat up to three times, then repeat the series once if needed. After eating spicy foods, take *Nux vomica*; after rich foods, take *Carbo vegetabilis;* and for burning pain, take *Arsenicum album.*

■ Hydrotherapy

Placing an ice pack over your stomach for five to 10 minutes before eating may help prevent an attack of heartburn. To relieve heartburn, drink charcoal slurry: Stir 1 tbsp charcoal powder (available at health food stores) into a 10-oz glass of water; let the black powder settle to the bottom of the glass and drink the slurry water on top. Keep in mind that charcoal can interfere with the body's absorption of any medications you may be taking at the time.

■ Nutrition and Diet

Certain foods commonly relax the LES, including tomatoes, citrus fruits, garlic, onions, chocolate, coffee, alcohol, and peppermint. Try to avoid these foods, as well as dishes high in fats and oils (animal or vegetable), which often lead to heartburn. In general, try to refrain from eating large meals;

Acupressure

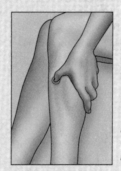

Stomach 36 • *To find this point, measure four finger widths below the kneecap just outside the shinbone. To verify the location, flex your foot; you should feel a muscle bulge at the point site. Apply steady pressure with a finger or thumb, then repeat on the other leg.*

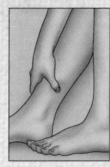

Spleen 6 • *Measure four finger widths up from the top of the right inside anklebone. With your thumb, press near the edge of the shinbone. Repeat on the other leg. (Do not use this point if you are pregnant.)*

---

instead, eat four or five small meals each day, and eat slowly. This, along with maintaining a weight in proportion to your height, will minimize abdominal pressure—and heartburn.

Prevention

Heartburn is often preventable. The keys are maintaining a reasonable weight, avoiding foods that cause stomach acid to reflux into your esophagus, getting adequate rest and exercise, and minimizing stress. Certain medications, especially some antibiotics and aspirin, can also lead to heartburn, so seek alternatives when possible.

Chew your food slowly and thoroughly, and avoid eating within two to three hours of bedtime. If you must lie down after eating, lie on your left side; your stomach is lower than your esophagus in this position. ■

OF SPECIAL INTEREST

The Milk Myth

Milk is not a remedy for heartburn. The soothing effect felt when drinking milk is deceiving; once in the stomach, milk's fat, calcium, and protein cause increased acid secretion and worsened heartburn. Mints are also often credited with alleviating heartburn, but they don't: Mint actually relaxes the lower esophageal sphincter, making heartburn more likely.

ℋemorrhoids

Symptoms

- Bright red anal bleeding that may streak the bowel movement or the toilet tissue.
- Tenderness or pain during bowel movements.
- Painful swelling or a lump near the anus.
- Anal itching.
- A mucous anal discharge.

Call Your Doctor If

- you experience any anal bleeding for the first time, even if you believe you have hemorrhoids. Colon polyps, colitis, Crohn's disease, and colorectal cancer can also cause anal bleeding. An accurate diagnosis is essential.
- you have been diagnosed with hemorrhoids and you have anal bleeding that is chronic (daily or weekly) or more profuse than the streaking described above. Although rare, excessive hemorrhoidal bleeding can cause anemia.

Hemorrhoids are essentially varicose veins of the rectum. The hemorrhoidal veins are located in the lowest area of the rectum and the anus. Sometimes they swell, so that the vein walls become stretched, thin, and irritated by passing bowel movements. When these swollen veins bleed, itch, or hurt, they are known as hemorrhoids, or piles. Hemorrhoids are classified into two general categories:

Internal hemorrhoids lie far enough inside the rectum that you can't see or feel them, and usually don't hurt. Bleeding may be the only sign of their presence. External hemorrhoids lie within the anus and are often painful. If an external hemorrhoid prolapses, or enlarges and protrudes outside the anal sphincter (usually in the course of passing a stool), you can see and feel it.

Hemorrhoids are the most common cause of anal bleeding and are rarely dangerous, but you must see your physician for a definite diagnosis.

Treatment Options

Most hemorrhoid treatments aim to minimize pain and itching. The efficacy of over-the-counter remedies, the basic ingredient of which is some form of lubricant, such as lanolin, is debatable; plain petroleum jelly often works just as well. Some remedies also contain an anesthetic to relieve pain. Creams or ointments are best; suppositories usually go too far up into the anal canal to help. The following remedies can also help alleviate hemorrhoid discomfort. If symptoms persist, contact your doctor.

▓ Acupuncture

Responsive points for relieving hemorrhoid pain are Stomach 36 *(see page 67)*, and Large Intestine 11 *(see page 49)*. A technique known as deep drainage can be extremely effective; see a licensed practitioner for this and other acupuncture treatments.

▓ Herbal Therapies

Applied twice daily, pilewort *(Ranunculus ficaria)* ointment can reduce the pain of external hemorrhoids: Simmer 2 tbsp fresh or dried pilewort in 7 oz petroleum jelly for 10 minutes. Allow to cool before using; store leftover ointment in a closed

Yoga

Shoulder Stand • *To encourage blood flow away from hemorrhoids and reduce pain, lie on your back and lift both legs until they are at a right angle to your back. Supporting your hips with your hands, push your back and legs upward until they are vertical. Slowly lower your legs to release.*

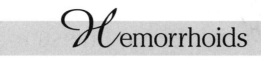emorrhoids

container. Pilewort may also be taken as a tea. Witch hazel *(Hamamelis virginiana)* applied to external hemorrhoids can also help.

Homeopathy
More than a dozen remedies, each taken at 12x, can help hemorrhoid pain. Choosing the right one requires attention to your symptoms and, usually, a homeopath's help. For a sore, bruised, and perhaps bleeding anus, try *Hamamelis. Aesculus* can ease sharp, spiking rectal pain that is worsened with bowel movements, and *Sulfur* can reduce burning and itching aggravated by warmth.

Hydrotherapy
Warm (not hot) sitz baths are often recommended for hemorrhoid discomfort: Sit in about three inches of warm water for 15 minutes, several times a day, especially after a bowel movement.

Massage
This technique moves matter through the intestines, helping to prevent the constipation that contributes to hemorrhoids. Begin on your left side. Lie on your back, raise your knees, and using your fingers or your palm to make long, sweeping strokes, stroke from a point just below your ribs toward your feet; then stroke across your abdomen from the right to left just below your rib cage. Finally, point your fingertips toward your feet, and drag your hand up your right side from pelvis to ribs. Repeat each stroke three to six times.

Nutrition and Diet
Prevent constipation by following a high-fiber diet. Meals and snacks should consist primarily of vegetables, fruit, nuts, and whole grains, and as few refined foods and meats as possible. If this is a big change for you, introduce the new foods slowly, to avoid gas. If you aren't able to eat enough high-fiber food, supplement your diet with psyllium stool softeners or bulk-forming agents. (Avoid laxatives, which cause diarrhea that can further irritate the swollen veins.) Drink up to eight glasses of fluid each day; if your life is especially active or if you live in a hot climate, you will need more.

Monitor your sodium intake. Excess salt in the diet causes fluid retention, which means swelling in all veins, including hemorrhoids.

Yoga
Yoga can encourage blood flow away from hemorrhoids, reducing pain, inflammation, and bleeding. Try the Shoulder Stand *(opposite)* and the Half Shoulder Stand *(see page 137)*, holding each posture for a few minutes each day. A good complement for these postures is lying on a slant board with your head down for 15 minutes daily.

Home Remedies

- Try not to sit for hours at a time, but if you must, take breaks: Once every hour, get up and move around for at least five minutes. A doughnut-shaped cushion can ease hemorrhoid pressure and pain.
- Insert petroleum jelly just inside the anus to make bowel movements less painful.
- Dab witch hazel *(Hamamelis virginiana)*, a soothing anti-inflammatory agent, on irritated hemorrhoids to reduce pain and itching.
- Bathe regularly to keep the anal area clean, but be gentle: Excessive scrubbing, especially with soap, can intensify irritation.
- Don't sit on the toilet for more than five minutes at a time, and when wiping, be gentle. If toilet paper is irritating, try dampening it first, or use cotton balls or alcohol-free baby wipes.
- When performing any task that requires exertion, be sure to breathe evenly. It's common to hold your breath during exertion, but if you do, you're straining, and contributing to hemorrhoid pain and bleeding.

Prevention

A healthful diet and lifestyle are good insurance for preventing hemorrhoids, whether you already suffer hemorrhoid symptoms or are intent on never having them. Regular exercise is also important, especially if you work a sedentary job. Exercise helps in several ways: It keeps weight down, makes constipation less likely, and enhances muscle tone. ∎

*H*igh Blood Pressure

Symptoms

In the vast majority of cases, there are no clear warning signs of hypertension (high blood pressure). If symptoms do occur, they may include:

- Headaches, chest pain or tightness, nosebleeds, and numbness and tingling; you may have severe hypertension.

- Excessive perspiration, muscle cramps, weakness, palpitations, and frequent urination; you may have secondary hypertension, possibly caused by kidney disease, a tumor, or an adrenal gland disorder.

Call Your Doctor If

- while taking antihypertensive drugs you experience worrisome side effects, such as drowsiness, constipation, dizziness, or loss of sexual function. Your doctor may need to prescribe a different drug.

- you are pregnant and develop hypertension; high blood pressure can affect not only your health but also that of your unborn child.

- you are experiencing severe headaches, blurred vision, nausea, and confusion or memory loss; you may have malignant hypertension, the name for hypertension that causes organ damage. Malignant hypertension can result in stroke or heart attack if left untreated.

- your diastolic pressure—the second number in a blood pressure reading—suddenly shoots above 130; you may have malignant hypertension.

Blood pressure—the force of blood pushing against artery walls as it courses through the body—naturally rises and falls with changes in activity or emotional state. It's also normal for blood pressure to vary from person to person, even from one area of your body to another. But when blood pressure remains consistently high, corrective steps should be taken.

Treatment Options

Many alternative therapies for high blood pressure focus on relaxation techniques. Others are attempts to get closer to the physiological roots of the problem, either by changing the patient's habits or lifestyle, or by influencing the operation of the heart and blood vessels.

Body Work
Regular sessions of massage or shiatsu can help lower blood pressure by promoting relaxation. Both therapies employ touch and manipulation to reduce tension in the body.

Chinese Medicine
Traditional Chinese healers treat high blood pressure by coupling acupuncture with herbal and massage therapy. Acupuncture may benefit people with moderate hypertension, but it is not recommended for those with severe cases. Chrysanthemum flower *(Chrysanthemum indicum),* peony *(Paeonia lactiflora)* root, eucommia *(Eucommia ulmoides)* bark, and prunella *(Prunella vulgaris)* are among the many Chinese herbs that might be prescribed in combination formulas for high blood pressure.

Herbal Therapies
Hawthorn *(Crataegus laevigata),* used to treat many circulatory disorders, may help reduce high blood pressure. Over time, the herb may help dilate blood vessels while also moderating heart rate. Hawthorn tea can be prepared at home by steeping the dried flowers and berries in hot water for 10 to 15 minutes. Research indicates that ample consumption of garlic *(Allium sativum)* and onion *(Allium cepa)* can help reduce blood pressure. Valerian *(Valeriana officinalis),* used only when need-

*H*igh Blood Pressure

ed, may work as a relaxant for people experiencing undue stress. *(See also Stress.)*

Mind/Body Medicine

A number of methods, including biofeedback, meditation, and hypnotherapy, call on the mind to relax the body and, practiced over time with guidance from trained professionals, may help lower blood pressure. Positive imagery—picturing yourself floating in calm water, for instance—can also work well for some people.

Nutrition and Diet

Adjusting the foods you eat will help keep your blood pressure in check. Your diet should be high in fiber and low in fat and salt. With these pointers in mind, emphasize fruits, vegetables, and whole grains. Enhance the flavor of your food with seasonings other than salt, and avoid processed foods, which tend to be high in sodium. You should also watch what you drink. Studies suggest that caffeine elevates blood pressure, at least temporarily, while moderate use of alcohol may lower it. But keep cocktails to a minimum; more than two ounces of alcohol per day can aggravate hypertension.

Of the vitamins and minerals that help lower blood pressure, potassium has one of the best track records. To get the 3,000 to 4,000 mg per day that researchers recommend, start eating more fresh vegetables and fruits, especially potatoes and bananas. According to several studies, daily doses of calcium (800 mg) or magnesium (300 mg) can help. Fish is a good source of fatty acids, which help relax arteries and thin the blood. Although it does contain sodium, celery is especially beneficial because it also contains ingredients believed to relax blood vessel walls.

Yoga

Mainly because of its relaxing effects, yoga is highly recommended for hypertension.

Home Remedies

- Adopt a healthful diet. Eat lots of fruit, vegetables, and whole grains. Give up salty foods and add seasonings other than salt to your meals. Go easy on alcohol and caffeine.

- Exercise regularly to shed extra pounds and get your blood flowing. Activities such as walking, jogging, cycling, and swimming lower blood pressure over the long term.
- If you smoke, quit.

Prevention

You can help keep your blood pressure at a healthful level and reduce your risk of heart disease by making a few changes in your lifestyle.

- Watch what you eat. Stay away from salt and fat, concentrating instead on foods that are high in fiber, calcium, and magnesium.
- Get plenty of exercise. Regular aerobic workouts condition the heart and keep blood vessels dilated and working properly, as do daily yoga and stretching exercises.
- If you are overweight, try to trim down. Even a small reduction can make a big difference.
- If you smoke, now is the time to stop. ■

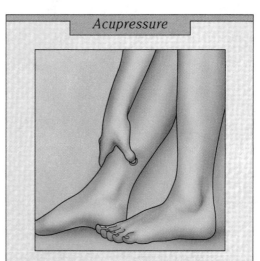

Acupressure

Spleen 6 • *Pressure on this point may help regulate blood pressure. The point is four finger widths up from the inner anklebone, near the edge of your shinbone. Press gently with your thumb for one minute, then switch legs. Do not use if you are pregnant.*

I

$\mathcal{I}$mmune Problems

Symptoms

In general, problems with your immune system manifest themselves as a tendency to catch colds, the flu, and various other infections more frequently than usual; to get easily tired; or to develop allergies. For specific symptoms of immune system disorders, see Allergies, Arthritis, Asthma, Chronic Fatigue Syndrome, and Hay Fever.

Call Your Doctor If

■ you suspect you have an immune system disorder; you need to be properly diagnosed so that you can be properly treated.

T he job of the immune system is to seek out, recognize, and destroy pathogens—disease-causing substances or organisms, such as bacteria and viruses. In fighting off these trespassers, your body produces such symptoms of illness as fever and malaise.

An overactive immune system results in autoimmune disorders. In these cases, for reasons that aren't clear, the immune system mistakes healthy tissues for foreign invaders and attacks them. Another type of immune error occurs when the system overreacts to something harmless, as with allergies. The opposite occurs when the immune system fails to respond adequately, resulting in immunodeficiency diseases such as AIDS.

For people who are generally healthy, the immune system can become temporarily depressed. When this happens, your body becomes more susceptible to infections, which hit you harder and stay with you longer than they would otherwise. A number of things can temporarily weaken the immune system, including environmental toxins, stress, poor diet, lack of exercise and sleep, and abuse of alcohol and tobacco.

Treatment Options

A number of alternative therapies are available for various autoimmune disorders. Consult the entries on multiple sclerosis, arthritis, and diabetes for possible remedies. The alternative choices suggested in the sections on allergies and hay fever may be helpful for those problems. Always seek the advice of a healthcare practitioner before embarking on alternative treatments.

In addition to the remedies below, you might want to try acupuncture, massage, or homeopathy, which may help with your specific symptoms. For each method, consult a specialist in the field.

■ Herbal Therapies
Echinacea (*Echinacea* spp.), long thought to be a potent immunostimulant, may have antiviral and antibacterial properties as well. Garlic *(Allium sativum)* may have anti-infective and immune-enhancing qualities. Mushrooms such as shiitake *(Lentinus edodes),* enokidake *(Flammulina velutipes),* and reishi *(Ganoderma lucidum)* may promote production of antibodies.

*I*mmune Problems

Various Chinese preparations may also be helpful: Dried slices of the remedy known as polyporus, from the mushroom *Polyporus umbellatus,* can be made into a tea and drunk for a tonic effect on the immune system. Astragalus *(Astragalus membranaceus)* tea or tincture may help combat viral infections and enhance the functioning of immune cells. The traditional *Xiao Chai Hu Wan* (Minor Bupleurum Pills) may strengthen the immune system. Asian Ginseng *(Panax ginseng)* may improve immune functioning by protecting against the damage caused by free radicals.

▓ Mind/Body Medicine
Research into the mind's effect on the immune system, called psychoneuroimmunology, has produced some findings on the relationship between happiness and health. One study has confirmed earlier reports that stress depresses immunity and that feeling good boosts it. Moreover, the data turned up an unexpected discovery: It seems that the impact of positive experiences such as expressions of love or feelings of accomplishment continues for two days, whereas the effects of negative events such as criticism or arguments last only one day. This suggests that the affirming consequences of happiness are more powerful and longer lasting than the negative effects of sadness—by 2 to 1.

Progressive relaxation techniques such as meditation, yoga, and qigong can promote a deep sense of relaxation and reduce stress. Regular exercise is considered to be another effective way to relieve stress.

▓ Nutrition and Diet
Nutritionists may recommend a diet high in fresh vegetables and fruit, whole grains, brown rice, low-fat dairy products, fish, and poultry, and low in refined sugars, white flour, junk foods, red meats, and saturated fats. A daily antioxidant multivitamin containing the U.S. recommended daily allowance of vitamins A, B complex, C, and E, with zinc, selenium, and other trace minerals, can play a role in shoring up immunity.

One theory holds that juice or water fasts may release a hormone that enhances the immune system. Fasts also cut down on the system's work load, because less energy is expended to process food allergens. Fasts are best attempted under the care of a doctor or nutritionist, who will advise you on how to safely begin and end one, as well as about some of the side effects to expect. Don't fast if you're pregnant or diabetic, or if you have a heart condition or an ulcer.

Prevention

- Avoid overeating and overindulging in alcohol, caffeine, and tobacco. Get plenty of rest, exercise regularly, and eat a balanced diet.
- Don't assault infections with antibiotics right away unless your physician deems it necessary. The immune system grows stronger with every battle won, so helping it fight with remedies less powerful than antibiotics—such as vitamins, homeopathic remedies, and herbal therapies—will allow the immune system to do its job.
- As much as possible, avoid radiation exposure, harmful chemicals, and prolonged use of immunosuppressive drugs such as corticosteroids, all of which can damage immunity. ■

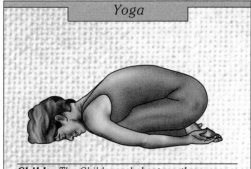

Yoga

Child • *The Child may help strengthen your immune system. Sit on your heels, thighs together. Exhale slowly while bending forward from your hips. Bring your forehead to the floor. Breathe deeply for 20 seconds, then inhale as you arise. Do this once, three or four times a day.*

I

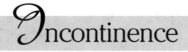

Incontinence

Symptoms

■ Inability to control urination.

■ Involuntary urination when coughing, laughing, sneezing, running, or performing other physical activity.

Call Your Doctor If

■ you have become unable to control your urination after an illness such as a bladder infection or after taking a new medication. Sudden loss of urinary control may also indicate neurological damage.

■ self-help remedies for controlling your urination are not working.

A lthough it is typically age related, incontinence—the involuntary loss of urine—is not, as is commonly believed, an inevitable consequence of aging. The condition often reflects an underlying disorder and is usually treatable, even in the elderly. With proper care, about 70 percent of cases can be improved or cured.

If left untreated, however, the condition will not improve and may actually worsen. Incontinence can lead to bladder or urinary tract infections. And the presence of leaked urine on the skin may cause uncomfortable rashes or other skin disorders. In those instances where treatment doesn't work, patients can avoid such complications by using special absorbent pads and other aids designed to help manage the problem.

Types of Incontinence

Medical professionals group incontinence into three major categories, although many people—women especially—experience symptoms of more than one. With stress incontinence, the muscles surrounding the urethra are so weakened that they can no longer resist a sudden increase in bladder pressure. Coughing, sneezing, laughing, exercising, or otherwise moving in a way that puts sudden pressure on the bladder can cause leakage—but usually only a few drops. With urge incontinence, the bladder, like that of an infant or toddler, simply contracts whenever it is full; the patient has no control over the sudden urge to void. Overflow incontinence occurs when a patient can no longer feel the sensation that signals when it is time to void. The bladder never empties normally and remains at least partially full; excess urine just spills out, usually in relatively small amounts.

Treatment Options

Most cases of incontinence can be cured or, at the very least, greatly improved with treatment. Many conventional practitioners routinely recommend two nonmedical approaches—Kegel exercises (opposite) and biofeedback—for patients suffering from stress incontinence. Bladder retraining is another useful technique. For seven days you keep a written record of how much you drink, how often

ℐncontinence
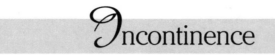

you urinate, and how much urine you produce. You then start urinating at scheduled intervals, usually every 30 or 60 minutes. Gradually, over a period of several weeks, you will increase the length of time between visits to the toilet.

If the condition persists or worsens, see a doctor for a full evaluation. Conventional approaches—including surgery—may be necessary.

Acupuncture
Acupuncturists believe that incontinence results from a deficiency of kidney and spleen chi. To restore the balance of chi in the affected parts, practitioners stimulate the specific points related to these organs and their channels. Consult a professional acupuncturist.

Biofeedback
Studies have shown that biofeedback techniques can lead to complete bladder control in up to 25 percent of incontinent patients and to substantial improvement in another 30 to 50 percent. Treatment sessions typically involve inserting a catheter through the urethra into the bladder and then slowly filling the bladder with fluid while the patient uses biofeedback techniques to control the urge to urinate.

Homeopathy
For stress incontinence, particularly in the elderly, try *Causticum,* which is said to restore vitality to aging tissue. For both stress and urge incontinence, particularly when a person is rising from a prone position, try *Pulsatilla,* thought to relieve irritation of the lining of the urinary tract system and restore it to proper functioning.

Nutrition and Diet
Try to keep your weight down. Excess weight puts pressure on bladder muscles, weakening them.

The straining that accompanies constipation can also weaken bladder muscles. Avoid constipation by increasing the fiber in your diet; eat more whole-grain foods and fruits and vegetables.

Avoid alcohol, caffeine, decaffeinated drinks, sugar and sugar substitutes, spicy foods, and acidic fruits and juices—all of which can irritate

the bladder and trigger leaks. Foods to which you are sensitive can also cause bladder irritation.

Home Remedies

- Double void: After urinating, wait a few seconds, then try again. Pouring cool water over the urinary opening after voiding can help.
- If you are a woman with stress incontinence, try crossing your legs when sneezing or coughing. This simple practice can be very effective in stopping leakage.
- Try bouncing on a minitrampoline for exercise; after several days, the pelvic floor muscles become strengthened enough to help prevent stress incontinence. ■

Kegel Exercises

Women with stress incontinence can use Kegel exercises to strengthen the pelvic floor muscles that support the uterus and bladder and control contractions of the vagina and urethra. While urinating, slowly contract the pelvic floor muscles, halting the flow of urine. Hold for up to 10 seconds and repeat several times. You can also do the exercises at other times, while standing, sitting, or lying down.

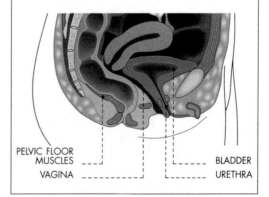

PELVIC FLOOR MUSCLES
VAGINA
BLADDER
URETHRA

I

$\mathcal{I}$ndigestion

Symptoms

- Heartburn.
- Gas or belching.
- Abdominal pressure and/or pain, which can radiate toward the chest.
- Mild nausea.
- Vomiting.

Call Your Doctor If

- any abdominal pain continues for more than six hours; this may indicate appendicitis, stomach ulcers, gallstones, or another serious problem or disease. You may need emergency care.
- you experience indigestion with any of the following: prolonged vomiting, vomiting of blood, black or bloody bowel movements, severe upper abdominal pain, pain radiating into your neck and shoulder, shortness of breath, or feeling weak or faint. Your indigestion may be part of a larger problem, such as gallstones, gastritis, pancreatic trouble, stomach ulcers, or possibly cancer. Or you might be having a heart attack; get medical help immediately.
- you have repeated bouts of indigestion accompanied by abdominal pain, fever, or dark urine. Your discomfort may indicate gallstones, stomach ulcers, or liver disease.
- your indigestion consistently follows your eating dairy products. You may suffer from lactose intolerance.

I ndigestion is a catchall term for assorted stomach discomforts. Symptoms of indigestion are cues that normal digestion has been interrupted for one or more reasons. If stomach acid enters the esophagus, for example, you may feel heartburn. Swallowing too much air while eating or drinking can induce a distended stomach and cause excessive belching. Stomach infections or inflammation can bring on gastritis. Sufferers of irritable bowel syndrome may regularly experience abdominal pain, bloating, and diarrhea.

Indigestion may be occasional or chronic (daily or almost daily). Though uncomfortable, indigestion itself is not life threatening. It can accompany serious problems, however, and should not be ignored.

Common Causes

Everyone—all ages, men and women alike—feels occasional indigestion. The likelihood increases with age as the digestive system gradually becomes less efficient. Occasional or chronic indigestion may be brought on by overeating; overindulging in alcohol; frequent use of analgesics—such as aspirin—and other pain relievers; eating while under stress; or eating food that does not agree with your system.

Two common causes of chronic indigestion are obesity, which increases pressure in the abdomen, and smoking, which increases the production of stomach acid and relaxes the sphincter between the esophagus and stomach. Overeating—even if it doesn't lead to obesity—is also a major cause of indigestion and of a general weakening of the digestive system. In addition, about half of all chronic indigestion sufferers are infected with the bacterium *Helicobacter pylori*. This bacterium is known to cause stomach ulcers, and researchers are trying to determine if it causes other kinds of indigestion as well.

Treatment Options

Because indigestion sufferers may have several disorders at once, healers suggest diverse therapies. Fortunately, there are many choices for relief. With most alternative treatments, patience is essential. Quelling persistent indigestion may take weeks or

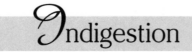

Indigestion

even months. Remember, however, that indigestion can result from a number of causes, so no single remedy will help everyone.

If it is determined that your indigestion is caused by *Helicobacter pylori,* you may need to see a doctor for a prescription of antibiotics to treat the infection.

Acupressure
To reduce symptoms of indigestion, massage the following for at least one minute: Large Intestine 4 *(see pages 65 and 117),* and Stomach 36 *(see page 67).* If gas is also a problem, add Spleen 6 *(see page 67).*

Aromatherapy
The essential oils of tarragon *(Artemisia dracunculus),* rosemary *(Rosmarinus officinalis),* and marjoram can reduce spasms of the digestive tract. Take 1 drop of one of these oils internally with either honey or a so-called carrier oil such as almond oil.

Ayurvedic Medicine
Shatavari may speed up digestion and alleviate many indigestion symptoms. Ayurveda bitters—including those from the trunk wood and bark of the common teak tree *(Tectona grandis)*—may also enhance digestion. Other remedies include infusions or powders made from mint, chamomile, and fennel seeds. Combined formulas include *Gasex* for adults (two to three tablets chewed after meals) and *Bonnisan* for children (consult a practitioner for dosages appropriate for the age of your child).

Herbal Therapies
Various teas may calm digestive distress. To reduce stomach acidity, drink meadowsweet *(Filipendula ulmaria)* tea once or twice daily, before meals (add 1 tsp to 1 cup boiling water, steep for 10 minutes, then filter). If you also feel stressed, add lavender *(Lavandula officinalis)* or chamomile *(Matricaria recutita).* If bloating or gas is a problem, try a tea of peppermint *(Mentha piperita),* chamomile, or lemon balm *(Melissa officinalis).*

Certain herbs are reputed to promote digestion and soothe and heal the esophagus, making them particularly appropriate for indigestion with

heartburn. About 30 minutes before eating, drink ½ cup of tea made from goldenseal *(Hydrastis canadensis),* barberry *(Berberis vulgaris)* bark, gentian *(Gentiana lutea)* root, or Oregon grape *(Mahonia aquifolium)* root.

A number of Chinese herbal formulas, including *Po Chai* and Pill Curing, are effective against certain types of acute indigestion. A practitioner of Chinese medicine can prescribe a remedy that's appropriate for your condition.

Hydrotherapy
Place a hot-water bottle over the abdomen after meals. A hot compress or moist abdominal bandage can also help relieve indigestion.

Massage
Gentle massage properly applied to the abdomen can help speed digestion and alleviate the discomfort of indigestion.

Home Remedies

- Refrain from smoking, especially before eating.
- Try one or several of the herbal teas above to relieve your specific symptoms.
- Relax after eating. Exercise diverts blood from the stomach, making digestion less efficient.
- If you frequently chew gum, stop for a while to see if your symptoms dissipate. It's common to swallow air when chewing gum, which can cause indigestion.

Prevention

Indigestion is universal; it's almost impossible to avoid it forever. You can encounter it less often, however, if you chew your food well, watch your weight, avoid overeating (especially foods rich in fat) or overindulging in alcohol, avoid your "trigger" foods, and abstain from smoking. ■

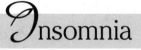 Insomnia

Symptoms

- Persistent trouble falling asleep.
- Failure to sleep through the night.
- Waking up earlier than usual.

Call Your Doctor If

- you experience disturbed sleep for more than a month without apparent cause. You may need referral to a sleep-disorder specialist to monitor your sleep patterns and test for underlying physical ailments.
- your insomnia is associated with a life-changing event, such as the loss of a job or a loved one. You may need sleep medication for a brief period.
- you never seem to get enough sleep and fall asleep without warning during the day. You may be suffering from narcolepsy.

 fter infancy, humans function the way the world turns—on a natural cycle that repeats itself about every 24 hours. During this daily cycle—which is known as the circadian rhythm—most adults sleep between six and eight hours, usually at night and without interruption. Although a few nights of poor sleep do no harm, prolonged insomnia can have serious consequences.

Insomnia can be described in terms of both duration and severity. Transient insomnia is associated with a temporary disturbance of one's normal sleeping pattern and usually lasts no more than several nights. Short-term insomnia, lasting two or three weeks, can accompany worry or stress and typically disappears when the apparent cause is resolved. Chronic insomnia is a more complex disorder with potentially serious effects.

Narcolepsy is characterized by attacks of irresistible drowsiness during the day, disrupting the pattern of a person's normal activity. A narcoleptic may not sleep well at night but suffer sleep attacks during the day.

Treatment Options

Many poor sleepers simply need help relaxing. If you're a habitual insomniac and trying to get to sleep just makes you feel more awake, the following remedies may help reduce your worry about sleep while relaxing your body and mind. If the root cause of insomnia is stress, any treatment must address the underlying problem.

Aromatherapy
A relaxant effect may be provided by oils of Roman chamomile *(Anthemis nobilis)*, lavender *(Lavandula angustifolia)*, neroli, rose, or marjoram. Add a few drops to your bathwater or sprinkle a few drops on a handkerchief and inhale.

Exercise
Moderate exercise—a 20- to 30-minute routine three or four times a week—will help you sleep better and give you more energy. Tailor the routine to your physical condition and exercise in the morning or afternoon, not close to bedtime. Breathing exercises can promote relaxation; here's a routine you can do anywhere, anytime:
- Exhale completely through your mouth.

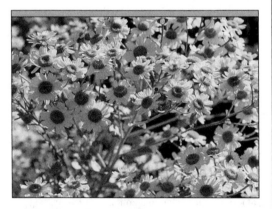

Chamomile • An herbal tea made from the flowers of the German chamomile (Matricaria recutita) plant can be very calming and soothing. You can buy prepared bags of chamomile tea or make your own by steeping 2 tsp flowers in 8 oz piping hot water for 10 minutes.

Insomnia

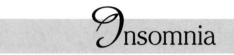

- Inhale through your nose to a count of four.
- Hold your breath for a count of seven.
- Exhale through your mouth for a count of eight. Repeat the cycle three times.

Herbal Therapies

Half an hour before bedtime, drink a calming herbal tea made with chamomile (Matricaria recutita), lime blossom (Tilia cordata), passionflower (Passiflora incarnata), or hops (Humulus lupulus); for insomnia from nervous tension, use vervain (Verbena officinalis) or skullcap (Scutellaria lateriflora). Valerian (Valeriana officinalis) is effective and seldom causes morning sleepiness: Brew valerian tea or take about 20 drops of tincture in water at bedtime; experiment to find the dosage that suits you best. Note that valerian, like any sleeping aid, acts as a central nervous system depressant and should not be used every night.

Homeopathy

For insomnia, a homeopathic practitioner may prescribe Nux vomica if the cause is anxiety or restlessness, Ignatia if the insomnia is related to grief, Coffea if it is related to excitability, or Muriaticum acidum if it stems from emotional problems.

Massage

Massage can promote relaxation and better sleep. While this may not be possible on a daily basis, it is a good complement to full-body exercises that may have caused stiff, tight muscles. Sessions with a massage therapist, or a massage routine performed by a partner, can be especially helpful when the insomnia is due to stress and anxiety, as well as muscular stiffness or discomfort.

Mind/Body Medicine

Meditation, yoga, and biofeedback can reduce tension and promote better sleep. Visualization, or guided imagery, may help you relax: Hold a peaceful image in your mind before bedtime.

Nutrition and Diet

Melatonin, a hormone secreted naturally by the pineal gland, is said to induce sleep without producing negative side effects; try a capsule nightly at bedtime for two weeks. The dosage should range anywhere from .3 to 1 mg. You may want to start by trying the lowest dose, which has proved effective with some people. Because experience with this hormone is limited, you may also want to consult your healthcare practitioner.

Calcium and magnesium taken 45 minutes before bedtime have a tranquilizing effect. Use a 1:1 ratio, in tablet or capsule form.

High or low blood sugar can disrupt sleep patterns. To help stabilize blood sugar, avoid sweets and fruit juices. To actuate the brain's sedative neurotransmitters, eat starchy food—a plain baked potato, a slice of bread, or an apple—half an hour before bedtime.

Warm milk, a traditional sleep aid, may provide a benefit that is more psychological than physiological. It does contain tryptophan, a sleep-inducing amino acid, but it also contains many other amino acids that compete to enter the brain.

Home Remedies

Be sure your bedroom is quiet and dark. Earplugs and eye masks may help; some light comes in even through closed eyelids.

Both children and adults may have trouble sleeping if they are overstimulated by activity or by watching television just before bedtime. A quarter-hour of quiet conversation, light reading, or soft music may make all the difference.

If you wake up at night and can't go back to sleep, remain quiet and relaxed. Sleep is normally punctuated by periods of restlessness, or even waking. Be patient; sleep usually returns.

Prevention

Try not to be rigid about when and how much you sleep. Worrying about a sleep schedule can just make it harder to fall asleep. If you prefer taking a nap during the day and sleeping less at night, do so. The total amount of sleep you get in 24 hours is more important than your daily schedule. ■

*I*rritable Bowel Syndrome

Symptoms

■ Constipation or diarrhea shortly after meals, over a period of several months, usually accompanied by abdominal cramps or bloating and increased intestinal gas.

■ Bowel movements different in frequency or consistency from your normal pattern.

Call Your Doctor If

■ you have pain in the lower left abdomen, fever, and a change in the frequency of bowel movements; you may have diverticulitis.

■ you discover blood in your stools; you could have colon polyps or colorectal cancer.

■ you have a fever, or you have been losing weight unexpectedly; such symptoms may signal disorders such as ulcerative colitis or Crohn's disease.

I *rritable bowel syndrome (IBS), which is sometimes referred to as spastic colon or spastic colitis, is the most common of all digestive disorders. The most frequently encountered symptom is abdominal pain with diarrhea or soft, frequent stools. In other cases, IBS comes with abdominal cramps and painful constipation, usually following meals. Whatever the specific symptoms, your digestion appears to be normal but your bowel movements become abnormal and stay that way for several weeks or longer. Irritable bowel syndrome affects 10 to 15 percent of adults at some time in their lives, often during periods of significant change or stress.*

Treatment Options

Various herbal and dietary remedies may be effective in preventing or soothing the discomfort of diarrhea and constipation. Relaxation techniques may be particularly effective in coping with stress-related aspects of the problem.

■ Acupuncture

An acupuncturist will determine an appropriate approach by asking you questions about stresses in your life that may be at the root of the problem. Treatment for IBS typically involves 10 to 12 sessions in which needles are inserted along the liver, spleen, and kidney meridians. For symptomatic relief of diarrhea, the acupuncturist will probably insert the needles near the navel and left knee. To treat a bad bout of diarrhea, the practitioner may employ moxibustion, in which heat is applied near the points, for quick relief.

■ Exercise

Walking at an aerobic pace for 20 to 30 minutes gets the heart pumping, stimulates the digestive process, and relaxes the body. Vigorous noncompetitive exercise is also recognized as an effective way of combating and controlling stress. (Competitive sports, however, can add to stress for many individuals.) Yoga *(see the illustration at left)* not only conditions the muscles and connective tissue but also is thought to tone the internal organs, including the digestive tract, and release excess tension from the body.

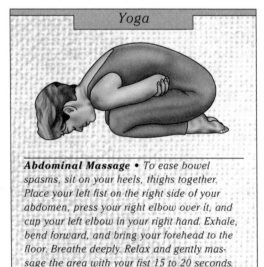

Yoga

Abdominal Massage • *To ease bowel spasms, sit on your heels, thighs together. Place your left fist on the right side of your abdomen, press your right elbow over it, and cup your left elbow in your right hand. Exhale, bend forward, and bring your forehead to the floor. Breathe deeply. Relax and gently massage the area with your fist 15 to 20 seconds. Rise and massage your abdomen with your fingers. Repeat on your left side. Do twice daily.*

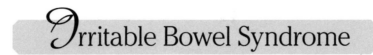

Irritable Bowel Syndrome

■ Herbal Therapies

For diarrhea, make a carob *(Ceratonia siliqua)* tea: Pour 1 cup hot water over 1 tsp roasted carob powder. Drink three times a day.

To calm an overactive gastrointestinal tract, try a European favorite: Take one or two enteric-coated peppermint *(Mentha piperita)* oil capsules between meals, three times daily. Reduce the dose if you have a burning sensation when you move your bowels. Another option is peppermint tea: Steep 1 tbsp dried peppermint leaves in a cup of boiling water for 30 minutes; drink three to four cups a day. Infusions of chamomile *(Matricaria recutita),* marsh mallow *(Althaea officinalis)* root, bayberry *(Myrica* spp.), or slippery elm *(Ulmus fulva)* also are soothing to the intestinal tract and can be made the same way.

■ Homeopathy

A homeopathic practitioner will determine which remedy is appropriate to get at the root cause of the IBS. For relief of occasional diarrhea, try prepared remedies available in health food stores. *Ignatia* may be helpful if you are having spasms of pain and diarrhea after emotional upsets. If you are passing offensive-smelling gas and mucus in the stools, take *Mercurius vivus.* If sudden cramplike pains are relieved by bending over, take *Colocynthis.* If your stools are soft but you have to strain to pass them, try *Nux vomica.*

■ Mind/Body Medicine

A number of techniques have been found helpful for IBS, including training in muscle relaxation. After four to six weeks of daily practice, you will learn how to relax your previously tense muscles and relieve symptoms brought on by stress.

Biofeedback training is another technique that has become accepted by more and more conventional doctors and often is covered by insurance. In one form of biofeedback, painless electrodes are placed on the forehead to monitor muscle tension as an indicator of stress. Patients are taught to relax their muscles by actuating audio or visual signals that indicate the level of tension in the muscle.

Of all the relaxation techniques, the most familiar may be hypnotherapy. A practitioner uses the power of suggestion to teach a patient in a hypnotic state how to relax the smooth muscles of the intestines. Guided imagery, often taught by yoga instructors and massage therapists, can also teach you new ways to relax yourself.

■ Nutrition and Diet

Certain foods may contribute to IBS by irritating your gastrointestinal tract. Most things that people say taste good—from hamburgers and fries to ice cream and chocolate—are made with lots of fat. Whether it's vegetable oil or animal fat, or saturated or unsaturated, dietary fat overload is something many people simply can't handle. Other known irritants to some people's digestive tracts are eggs and dairy products, spicy foods, and stimulants, including caffeinated beverages and white sugar; decaffeinated beverages are also a problem, as are other forms of sugar such as molasses, corn syrup, and fructose.

If you are like most Americans, you are not eating enough fiber. To correct a dietary fiber imbalance:

- gradually increase the amount of fresh fruits and vegetables, whole grains, and bran in your diet, or
- take 1 tbsp bran stirred into a glass of fruit juice or water every day, or
- take soluble fiber, like psyllium *(Plantago psyllium)* seed. Stir 1 tbsp into a glass of cold water and drink once a day. When you are taking supplemental fiber, be sure to drink several extra glasses of plain water a day. You may experience a certain amount of intestinal gas at first, but it should subside as your body adjusts to the new regimen.

Prevention

Healthy outlets for stress are great preventives to many gastrointestinal problems, including IBS. Get regular exercise—anything from a brisk 20-minute walk to a round of golf or tennis or a half-hour's worth of swimming laps. And take 10 minutes twice a day to just relax and let go of tensions. ■

Laryngitis

Symptoms

- Hoarseness and loss of voice.
- Pain when speaking.
- Tickling and rawness in the throat.
- A constant need to clear the throat.
- Loss of voice that is accompanied by the flu, a cold, or pneumonia.
- Fever (occasionally).

Call Your Doctor If

- hoarseness and discomfort last more than a week; this could signal a bacterial infection or a more serious disorder.
- you develop laryngitis after being exposed to environmental toxins, such as poisonous fumes or noxious odors; such exposure might have caused more damage than just a simple inflammation of your vocal cords.
- laryngitis occurs along with or as a result of alcohol abuse or chronic bronchitis, both of which require a doctor's care.
- a child's hoarseness turns into a sharp, barking cough, which could indicate a severely restricted airway or, possibly, croup.

Echinacea • *This attractive plant, known by gardeners as purple coneflower, is valued by herbalists for its roots. Echinacea root has antibacterial, antiviral, and immune-boosting properties that help wipe out the illness causing laryngitis.*

I *f you lose your voice, or if the sounds coming out of your mouth sound higher or lower than normal, you may have laryngitis. Specifically, this disorder is an inflammation of the mucous membrane of the larynx, or the part of your windpipe that contains the vocal cords. Your vocal cords open and close during the course of normal speech (right). If they become swollen, perhaps as a result of a viral or bacterial infection, overuse, or in some cases, an allergic reaction to a certain food, the sounds you make become distorted. You'll be hoarse, or you may lose your voice.*

Treatment Options

Viral laryngitis usually goes away by itself in a few days, so a persistent case is a warning sign that something other than a virus may be causing your symptoms. To treat laryngitis, alternative practitioners often prescribe methods to soothe the raw throat or boost the immune system.

Acupuncture
A recent study found that many patients with laryngitis or tonsillitis benefited from acupuncture. Consult a licensed acupuncturist for treatment.

Aromatherapy
The essential oils of thyme *(Thymus vulgaris)*, cypress, rosemary *(Rosmarinus officinalis)*, and sage can help relieve the discomfort of laryngitis; place a few drops on a handkerchief and inhale.

Ayurvedic Medicine
An Ayurvedic physician may recommend one of the following remedies for laryngitis: an infusion or powder of cloves or of the fruit of beleric myrobalan, an infusion of ginger or mint, a milk decoction or powder of licorice root.

Chinese Medicine
For acute laryngitis, a practitioner of Chinese medicine may prescribe *Hou Yan Wan,* or Throat Inflammation Pills (also known as Laryngitis Pills).

Herbal Therapies
To help restore the voice, try gargling with a tea made from red sage *(Salvia officinalis* var. *rubia),*

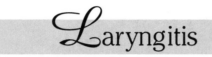 Laryngitis

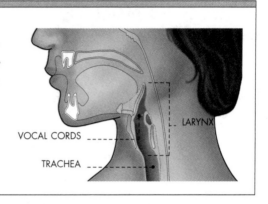

The Larynx and Voice Loss

The vocal cords are two taut bands that stretch across the larynx—a boxlike chamber at the upper part of the trachea, or windpipe. Air passing through these bands causes vibrations that produce sounds, which are shaped and modified by the tongue, teeth, and lips into speech. When the vocal cords are inflamed or infected because of laryngitis, the voice typically becomes hoarse or muted.

VOCAL CORDS

LARYNX

TRACHEA

bayberry (*Myrica* spp.), or white oak (*Quercus alba*) bark. A tincture of echinacea (*Echinacea* spp.) every hour for two days is thought to help boost the immune system. Mix 10 drops of the tincture in a glass of water and swallow.

■ Homeopathy

If laryngitis is a result of overuse or trauma to the vocal cords, use *Arnica* (6x or 12x) every hour; if you notice no improvement after four or five hours, try another preparation. For laryngitis that is accompanied by dryness of the throat and the feeling of a plug in the larynx, use *Spongia tosta* (12x) four times a day. For laryngitis accompanied by a dry, croupy cough that comes on suddenly after exposure to cold weather or with the first signs of a cold, use *Aconite* (6x or 12x) every two hours. If these remedies don't work, consult a practitioner.

■ Hydrotherapy

To soothe the discomfort of laryngitis, use a heating compress, which goes on cold but heats up as the body responds to the treatment.

Begin by placing a warm washcloth on your neck for two or three minutes. Soak a long, wide cotton cloth in cold water, then wring it out thoroughly and wrap it loosely around your neck. Next, wrap wool flannel (a wool scarf works nicely) around the cotton and secure it with a safety pin. Leave the compress in place for at least 30 minutes, preferably overnight. Follow the treatment with a quick cold sponge to the area. Change the compress every eight hours and allow the skin to dry for at least an hour between treatments.

■ Nutrition and Diet

Drinking plenty of fluids, eating lots of raw fruits and vegetables, and reducing your intake of refined carbohydrates may help speed your recovery from laryngitis. To boost your immune system, supplement your daily diet with 1,000 to 3,000 mg vitamin C, 10,000 to 20,000 IU of beta carotene (*vitamin A*), and garlic.

Home Remedies

- Rest your body as well as your voice—completely. If you must speak, whisper; do not engage the vocal cords at all.
- Drink plenty of liquids, such as water or tea mixed with a little honey or lemon.
- Inhale steam from a pot of boiling water.
- Apply warm compresses to your throat.

Prevention

To prevent laryngitis, avoid straining your voice and give it proper rest after overuse. If you're prone to laryngitis, try to stay away from cigarette smoke or other environmental toxins. If you think your laryngitis stems from an allergy to a certain kind of food, experiment by removing suspected items from your diet, then reintroduce them one by one while monitoring the effect. *(See Allergies.)* ■

$\mathcal{M}$enopause

Symptoms

Not all women experience symptoms with the onset of menopause. If symptoms occur, they may include:

- Hot flashes—sudden reddening or heating of the face, neck, and upper back, which may produce sweating. Flashes typically last only a few minutes.

- Night sweats, which may disrupt sleep and lead to insomnia.

- Pain during intercourse, caused by thinning of vaginal tissues and loss of lubrication.

- Increased nervousness, anxiety, or irritability.

- The need to urinate more often than before, especially during the night.

Call Your Doctor If

- you experience bleeding after menopause; among other possibilities, it may be a sign of uterine cancer, so you should be checked by your doctor.

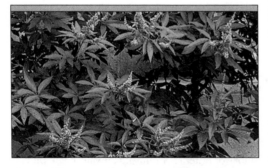

Chaste Tree • Used for centuries to manipulate the functioning of the female reproductive system, chaste tree can help relieve premenstrual syndrome and counter symptoms of menopause.

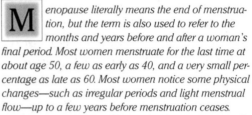

M *enopause literally means the end of menstruation, but the term is also used to refer to the months and years before and after a woman's final period. Most women menstruate for the last time at about age 50, a few as early as 40, and a very small percentage as late as 60. Most women notice some physical changes—such as irregular periods and light menstrual flow—up to a few years before menstruation ceases.*

As a woman ages, her ovaries slow and eventually cease their normal functions, including egg production. Even more significant, they decrease their production of estrogen and progesterone. As levels of these hormones—especially estrogen—decline, they cause changes throughout the body and particularly in the reproductive system, the most notable change being the end of menstruation. Decreased estrogen levels may also be responsible for the various symptoms associated with menopause, such as hot flashes and mood swings, which may or may not be present.

Some symptoms, including hot flashes and mood swings, are temporary and will pass as the body adjusts. But more serious problems can also result. Decreased levels of estrogen, for example, affect the way bones absorb calcium and can raise cholesterol levels in the blood; postmenopausal women thus face increased risk for developing both osteoporosis and cardiovascular diseases such as atherosclerosis.

Treatment Options

The most common approach to treating menopausal problems is to make up for the body's reduced production of estrogen. Known in conventional medicine as hormone replacement therapy, this technique is somewhat controversial because of certain side effects, so you should weigh the risks and benefits in consultation with your doctor.

Aromatherapy
Essential oils of clary sage *(Salvia sclarea)*, sage, and geranium can help ease the symptoms of menopause. Put a few drops in the bath, or sprinkle the oil on a handkerchief and inhale.

Ayurvedic Medicine
Depending on your needs, an Ayurvedic physician may recommend the combined formula *Geriforte* or

Menopause

one of the following: the powder of *shatavari* root, boiled in milk to which clarified butter (ghee) has been added, taken three times daily; or the powder of Indian nut grass, steeped in a pint of water and taken with ginger and honey three times a day.

Body Work

Many women find relief of menopausal symptoms through therapeutic touch, a method in which a healer holds his or her hands near the patient's body to sense and correct energy blockages. Consult a practitioner trained in this technique.

Herbal Therapies

A variety of herbs and foods may help relieve symptoms of menopause. Extracts and teas made from black cohosh *(Cimicifuga racemosa)* may supply beneficial amounts of phytoestrogen, or plant estrogen. Combinations of chaste tree *(Vitex agnuscastus),* motherwort *(Leonurus cardiaca),* wild yam *(Dioscorea villosa),* and other herbs may help reduce the frequency and discomfort of hot flashes, and may also relieve other symptoms. The herb horsetail *(Equisetum arvense),* thought to increase the absorption of calcium in the bones, may help prevent loss of bone density after menopause.

Some Chinese herbs—including dong quai *(Angelica sinensis)* and Asian ginseng *(Panax ginseng)*—may have estrogenic effects. Exact proportions are important, and some dosages are toxic; consult an herbalist. For hot flashes and night sweats, a Chinese medicine practitioner may recommend the formulas *Zhi Bai Ba Wei Wan* (Eight Flavor Pills) or *Liu Wei Di Huang Wan* (Six Flavor Pills).

Hydrotherapy

For relief from hot flashes, try a cold compress: Wet a cotton washcloth with ice water. Wring it out and apply it to the neck and chest. Hold the cloth in place for three minutes, rewetting it as needed to keep it cold. Dry the area after the treatment.

Mind/Body Medicine

Regardless of your religious affiliation or particular set of spiritual beliefs, prayer and meditation can be powerful tools to help you cope with the symptoms of menopause.

OF SPECIAL INTEREST

Menopausal Myths and Facts

Myth: *Menopause makes women emotionally unstable.*
Fact: *Most women experience no emotional problems; those that occur can be treated.*

Myth: *Menopause puts an end to sexual desire.*
Fact: *Vaginal dryness can make intercourse painful, reducing desire, but this is readily treated with vaginal lubricants or estrogen creams. Menopause itself can affect libido either positively or negatively; some women actually have increased libido with menopause.*

Myth: *Menopause disrupts a woman's life.*
Fact: *Most women experience few or no menopausal problems; 25 percent have moderate, treatable symptoms. In countries where age is respected, women report the fewest symptoms during menopause.*

Nutrition and Diet

Eating foods high in plant estrogens, such as soybeans and lima beans, may alleviate symptoms; additional sources include whole grains, other beans, nuts, and seeds.

Sound Therapy

A number of sound-healing and music-therapy techniques can be useful in treating the stress and other symptoms associated with menopause. Consult a music therapist or sound healer for a program that's right for you.

Home Remedies

- Raise your intake of calcium and magnesium and engage in weight-bearing exercises to avoid osteoporosis and maintain general good health.
- Take 400 to 800 IU of vitamin E daily to treat hot flashes and reduce the risk of cardiovascular disease.

$\mathcal{M}$enstrual Problems

Symptoms

- Menstruation does not occur. Called amenorrhea, this can come from pregnancy, overexercise, or anorexia nervosa.

- Menstruation is painful and produces clots. Called dysmenorrhea, this may be entirely normal, but it may also be caused by endometriosis; polyps, fibroids, or other lesions of the uterus; or an intrauterine device (IUD).

- Menstrual flow is heavy. Called menorrhagia, this can be a result of stress, endometriosis or other pelvic lesions, pelvic infection, or an IUD.

Call Your Doctor If

- you have heavy menstrual flow that fills a tampon or sanitary napkin within an hour; heavy flow can cause anemia.

- you have missed a period and think you may be pregnant; a late flow that is unusually heavy could indicate a miscarriage.

- you experience sharp abdominal pain before periods or during intercourse; you could have endometriosis.

- you get your period after menopause.

M *enstruation is a normal part of a woman's reproductive cycle. When an ovary releases an egg, it also releases the hormone estrogen, which stimulates the lining of the uterus to grow and engorge with blood. If the egg is not fertilized, the ovary releases progesterone, which makes the uterus shed its lining; the resulting menstrual flow typically consists of a few tablespoonfuls of blood and tissue fragments. This series of events repeats on a cycle of approximately 28 days until it is interrupted by pregnancy or ended by menopause.*

The degree of discomfort or pain a period causes, as well as the amount of menstrual flow, varies widely among individuals. Also, your own period may occasionally be heavier or more painful than usual. Such problems, while unpleasant, generally do not signal underlying disease. But you should be aware that the same complaints can sometimes indicate more serious conditions, such as endometriosis or an ovarian cyst.

The three main categories of menstrual irregularities are lack of period (amenorrhea), painful periods (dysmenorrhea), and heavy periods (menorrhagia). The following text explains these problems and what you can do about them.

LACK OF PERIOD

Although often no cause for concern, amenorrhea can be a sign of an underlying problem. It might indicate, for example, that you have low levels of estrogen in your system and are therefore at a greater risk of developing osteoporosis. Or it may signal a lack of progesterone and that you are at a greater risk for endometrial problems, including endometrial cancer. Also, of course, if you do not menstruate, you cannot become pregnant.

The lack of a period in a woman who has not yet begun to menstruate is known as primary amenorrhea; in a woman who has temporarily stopped menstruating, it is known as secondary amenorrhea. Primary amenorrhea has several causes, the most likely of which is that a girl has simply not yet reached puberty. (It is perfectly normal for puberty to occur as late as the age of 17.) But delayed puberty in a girl who is very thin or who exercises excessively is worrisome, because it could be an indication of anorexia nervosa; women

Menstrual Problems

who have very low body fat do not menstruate.

Primary amenorrhea can also point to other problems. In rare cases, for example, a girl might actually lack ovaries or a uterus and therefore not be able to menstruate. Or a tumor, an injury or trauma, or a structural defect might be interfering with some aspect of the menstrual cycle, from the production of hormones to the actions of the organs and tissues that the hormones affect.

Secondary amenorrhea can also be traced to injuries or structural abnormalities; one common cause is ovarian cysts. But factors such as stress can also disrupt the balance of hormones and thereby interrupt the normal cycle. Also, as in adolescence, extreme underweight can stop menstruation; if your period stops while you are dieting or in athletic training, you may be overdoing it. And, of course, amenorrhea could signal the onset of menopause or pregnancy.

PAINFUL PERIODS

Menstrual pain, or dysmenorrhea, is hardly unusual and in most cases is completely normal, even if troublesome. But there are situations in which painful periods may signal a condition that requires further evaluation by your doctor. And if your pain interferes with your normal activities, you should consider some of the treatments listed here, which may help bring you relief.

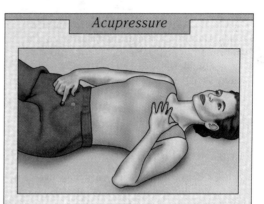

Acupressure

Conception Vessel 4 • *You may be able to correct irregular periods by working this point. Measure four finger widths down from your navel. Press your index finger firmly into your abdomen and hold for one to two minutes. Do this twice a day every day.*

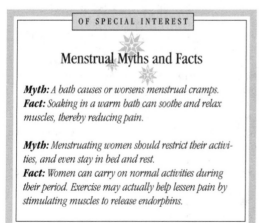

OF SPECIAL INTEREST

Menstrual Myths and Facts

Myth: *A bath causes or worsens menstrual cramps.*
Fact: *Soaking in a warm bath can soothe and relax muscles, thereby reducing pain.*

Myth: *Menstruating women should restrict their activities, and even stay in bed and rest.*
Fact: *Women can carry on normal activities during their period. Exercise may actually help lessen pain by stimulating muscles to release endorphins.*

If you have always had painful periods, they are probably the result of hormonal changes during your menstrual cycle. The factor most likely to be causing pain is that your body is producing an excess of prostaglandins—hormonelike substances that cause contractions of the uterus during menstruation and when a woman goes into labor. During menstruation, these contractions ensure that all the menstrual blood and tissue are expelled from the body, but excess prostaglandins can cause repeated contractions—and perhaps even spasms—which are experienced as cramping. It is common for these pains to persist throughout your reproductive years, but many women find that menstrual cramps become milder after they have had a baby.

Dysmenorrhea may, however, also be caused by an underlying condition, such as endometriosis, an infection, or growths in the uterus.

HEAVY PERIODS

A heavy period (menorrhagia) is a menstrual flow that lasts longer than eight days, saturates tampons or napkins within an hour, or includes large

CONTINUED

*M*enstrual Problems

clots of blood. Heavy periods may be caused by various factors—a hormonal imbalance, endometriosis, a pelvic infection, uterine growths such as fibroids, or use of an IUD. Excessive bleeding may signal other irregularities in your cycle: lack of ovulation, low levels of progesterone, or an excess of prostaglandins. Heavy periods can cause iron deficiency anemia.

Treatment Options

Treatment for primary amenorrhea may involve no more than waiting to see if nature takes its course. For a girl who exercises strenuously or who is very thin, a healthcare professional may advise a lighter training regimen or an effort to gain weight. Treatment for anorexia nervosa might also be necessary. For secondary amenorrhea, if you think stress is to blame, take steps to reduce stress in your life; this alone may restore your cycle.

Most of the alternative therapies for menstrual cramps focus on promoting the relaxation of tense muscles or on reducing tension in general. Treatment for menorrhagia (heavy periods) may include iron and folic acid supplements to treat and prevent anemia.

In addition to the suggestions listed below, see the appropriate entries for treatment advice related to an underlying condition.

Acupressure

An acupressure technique that may prove effective in correcting irregular menstrual periods is illustrated on page 87. For relief of pain associated with menstrual cramps, use the point known as Spleen 6 *(see page 67).*

Both acupressure and acupuncture use techniques that rely on spleen points to help control blood flow. See a practitioner for points and techniques to relieve excessive menstrual flow.

Aromatherapy

For painful periods, massage the lower abdomen, back, and legs with oil or lotion containing German chamomile *(Matricaria recutita).*

Practitioners of aromatherapy find that oils of geranium, juniper, and cypress, rubbed on the ab-

domen, may bring relief for sufferers of heavy menstrual flow.

Chiropractic

Chiropractic techniques can sometimes help relieve menstrual cramps; see a chiropractor for treatment.

Herbal Therapies

To help initiate menstrual flow, make a tincture of one part chaste tree *(Vitex agnus-castus),* two parts blue cohosh *(Caulophyllum thalictroides),* and two parts mugwort *(Artemisia argyi)* leaf; take 2 ml three times daily until menstrual flow begins.

To relieve cramps, drink a hot tea of 2 tsp cramp bark *(Viburnum opulus)* simmered for 15 minutes in 1 cup water; use this three times a day. Bilberry *(Vaccinium myrtillus)* and bromelain will also relax muscles. Dong quai *(Angelica sinensis)* and feverfew *(Tanacetum parthenium)* can relax uterine muscles; feverfew may work by inhibiting prostaglandin synthesis. Valerian *(Valeriana officinalis)* helps relax cramping muscles; however, it may be addictive and should be used only for a limited time. Consult an herbalist.

Evening primrose *(Oenothera biennis)* oil applied over painful areas can bring relief, but don't use it if there's a chance you may get pregnant. A castor-oil pack placed over painful areas can also be helpful.

Tension, anxiety, and painful spasms may be relieved with treatments of black haw *(Viburnum prunifolium),* skullcap *(Scutellaria lateriflora),* and black cohosh *(Cimicifuga racemosa).* Take equal parts of these herbs in 5-ml doses as needed.

Tea made from yarrow *(Achillea millefolium)* may help control bleeding associated with heavy periods. You may also benefit from taking a tincture made of equal parts life root *(Senecio aureus),* shepherd's purse *(Capsella bursa-pastoris),* and wild cranesbill *(Geranium maculatum);* take it twice daily in 5-ml doses.

A number of Chinese herbal formulas can help with menstrual problems. For a painful period, try the combination formula *Xiao Yao Wan* (Free and Easy Wanderer Pills); for excessive bleeding, *Yun Nan Bai Yao* may offer relief. See a practitioner of Chinese medicine for a diagnosis.

*M*enstrual Problems

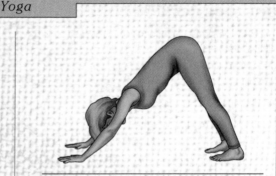

Yoga

Camel • *Performing this position regularly may help relieve amenorrhea or painful periods. First, kneel down. Lean backward as you exhale, placing your palms on the soles of your feet and tilting your head back (above). Inhale as you squeeze your buttocks and press your pelvis forward. Breathe slowly and hold this position for 20 seconds.*

To release, exhale as you sit back on your heels. Then inhale as you bring your body up, raising your head last. Breathe slowly and relax for 20 seconds. Do once or twice a day.

Downward Dog • *This pose helps release pelvic tension. From the Table position on your hands and knees, inhale and raise your pelvis to form an inverted V with your knees slightly bent.*

Press your palms and heels into the floor as you breathe deeply, keeping your arms and shoulders open and your back and legs straight (above). Hold for 20 to 30 seconds. To release, exhale as you resume the Table position. Sit back on your heels, bring your head up, and relax before attempting to stand up again. Do this two or three times a day.

■ Nutrition and Diet

To address nutrient deficiencies that may be causing amenorrhea, take supplements of or eat foods rich in zinc (fish, poultry, lean meats) and vitamin B complex (brewer's yeast, wheat germ).

Eating a balanced diet consisting of small meals throughout the day rather than three larger meals and avoiding sugar, salt, and caffeine may help relieve or prevent cramping. You may get relief from a multivitamin-multimineral supplement containing vitamin B complex, calcium, and magnesium. You can also take 50 mg of vitamin B_6 twice a day. Because your goal is to keep your body relaxed, avoid caffeine and other stimulants.

■ Yoga

Poses for relaxation and the relief of cramps are described and illustrated in the box above.

Home Remedies

- Take extra calcium and magnesium to stop uterine muscle cramps and to lessen the flow.
- Take a warm, relaxing bath.
- Drink herbal teas containing yarrow to help control bleeding.
- Apply a castor-oil pack to the abdomen to relax the muscles and lessen the flow.

Prevention

Maintain normal weight for your build, which helps prevent excess fat and estrogens in the body. Overweight women tend to have abnormal menstrual periods, perhaps because of an increase in estrogen-secreting cells.

Take a multivitamin-multimineral supplement including vitamins A, B complex, C, and E, as well as calcium and iron. ■

Mononucleosis

Symptoms

The early symptoms of mononucleosis resemble those of the flu, including:

- Severe fatigue.
- Headache.
- Sore throat, sometimes very severe.
- Chills, followed by a fever.
- Muscle aches.

After a day or two, the following symptoms may appear:

- Swollen lymph nodes, especially in the neck, armpits, or groin.
- Jaundice (a yellow tinge to the skin and eyes).
- Bruiselike areas inside the mouth.
- Soreness in the upper left abdomen (from an enlarged spleen).

Call Your Doctor If

- you have these symptoms, particularly for longer than 10 days, or if you have a severe sore throat for more than a day or two; you need to be examined by a doctor to rule out other illnesses.

- you develop swollen lymph nodes all over your body, which may be a sign of tuberculosis, cancer, or human immunodeficiency virus.

- you develop abdominal pain, which may indicate a ruptured spleen. Seek emergency medical treatment immediately.

CAUTION

If you have mononucleosis, avoid the risk of rupturing your spleen by forgoing any strenuous exercise until you have fully recovered.

M ononucleosis, often referred to as mono, is a very common viral illness. About 90 percent of people over age 35 have antibodies to mono in their blood, which means that they have been infected with the disease, probably during early childhood. When mono strikes young children, the illness is usually so mild that it passes for a common cold or the flu. When it occurs during adolescence or adulthood, however, the disease can be much more serious. Most people who come down with mono feel much better within two or three weeks. But sometimes the disease lingers for a year or so, causing recurrent, but successively milder, attacks.

Treatment Options

Most people recover on their own without any treatment within two weeks. Practitioners of alternative medicine recommend rest and various treatments to help relieve the symptoms of the disease. They also offer remedies to help strengthen the body's immune system.

Aromatherapy

Lavender (*Lavandula angustifolia*), bergamot, and eucalyptus globulus (*E. globulus*) are sometimes recommended to relieve fatigue and other symptoms of mono. Add a few drops of the essential oils of one or more of these herbs to a warm bath.

Chinese Medicine

The Chinese herbal formula *Xiao Chai Hu Wan* (Minor Bupleurum Pills) is often prescribed for the treatment of mononucleosis; it helps the liver clear infections from the body. Acupuncture may also be beneficial; consult a practitioner of Chinese medicine for dosages and treatment.

Herbal Therapies

To help fight the infection, try echinacea (*Echinacea* spp.) in glycerin tincture form; use 15 drops two times a day. To reduce the fever associated with mono, try drinking a tea made from elder (*Sambucus nigra*) flowers or yarrow (*Achillea millefolium*). Drink either tea three times a day. Or if you prefer, take 2 to 4 ml of the tincture of either herb three times a day.

To help cleanse the lymphatic system, try a

*M*ononucleosis

tea made from cleavers (*Galium* spp.) or wild indigo *(Baptisia tinctoria)*; drink three times a day. Alternatively, take 2 to 4 ml of tincture of cleavers or 1 ml of tincture of wild indigo three times daily.

To help with the anxiety and depression that sometimes accompany long-term bouts with mono, try St.-John's-wort *(Hypericum perforatum)* or vervain *(Verbena officinalis)*. Both herbs, when taken internally, appear to act as mild sedatives. Vervain is also recommended for jaundice, one of the symptoms of mono. Make a tea out of either herb and drink three times daily. Or take in tincture form: 1 to 4 ml of St.-John's-wort or 2 to 4 ml of vervain three times a day.

■ Homeopathy
Mononucleosis calls for a constitutional treatment—a set of remedies prescribed specifically for you, based on your symptoms and your medical history. Consult an experienced homeopath for such a treatment.

■ Mind/Body Medicine
Various relaxation techniques, such as meditation, biofeedback, and guided imagery, can be helpful in reducing stress, which can exacerbate the fatigue associated with mononucleosis.

■ Nutrition and Diet
To strengthen your immune system and help speed your recovery, eat plenty of whole (not processed) foods, especially fresh fruits and vegetables. Avoid foods that are high in saturated fats, animal proteins, and sugars, as they are difficult to digest and put stress on your body. Also avoid both caffeinated and decaffeinated beverages, which may weaken the immune system.

To maintain a better balance of blood sugar, and thus a more even energy level, eat four to six small meals throughout the day rather than three larger ones; try not to overeat at any one meal. Some people also find that eating a small portion of low-fat protein immediately on awakening in the morning and again in the evening before going to bed can help raise energy levels. Good choices of protein for this purpose include low-fat cheese as well as tofu, lentils, and other legumes.

Vitamin supplements may also enhance your immune system. Take vitamin A (2,500 to 10,000 IU daily), vitamin C (500 to 2,000 mg daily), and vitamin B complex (50 mg a day). You may also wish to try daily magnesium (200 to 500 mg), calcium (200 to 500 mg), and potassium aspartate (50 to 200 mg) supplements. Research has shown that these supplements can dramatically improve energy levels after six weeks of constant use.

■ Yoga
Yoga can help reduce fatigue. The exercises are gentle enough to be done even by someone with the illness. One recommended pose is the Cobra *(see page 38).*

Home Remedies

- Rest your body. Do not plan to return to your normal activity level for at least a month.
- Drink plenty of liquids to prevent dehydration.
- For sore throat, use a saline gargle—½ tsp salt in a glass of warm water.
- To help ease fatigue, massage your kidneys daily. With loose fists, rub your lower back for three to five minutes. A good occasion to do this is in the shower with warm water running down your back. ■

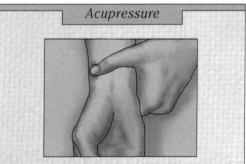

Acupressure

Lung 7 • *Pressing this point may bolster immunity and lung function. The point is located on the thumb side of the inner forearm, two finger widths above the crease in the wrist. Apply steady, firm pressure for one minute, then repeat on the other arm.*

$\mathcal{M}$otion Sickness

Symptoms

■ Sweating, dizziness, pallor, and nausea—sometimes leading to vomiting—while traveling by car, bus, train, ship, or airplane.

Call Your Doctor If

■ you are planning a trip and are concerned that you will be bothered by motion sickness that does not respond to alternative remedies; your doctor may prescribe antinausea drugs.

T *he nausea and dizziness that afflict some people when they are traveling in a vehicle certainly cause discomfort, but they are not serious. The symptoms of motion sickness usually subside either once your body adjusts to your mode of travel or shortly after the trip ends. Motion sickness may occur because your brain is receiving conflicting information from your sensory organs.*

Treatment Options

If you are prone to motion sickness, preparations for any trip should include measures to prevent the disorder or mechanisms to cope with it.

Acupressure
Much scientific research exists to substantiate the use of wrist point Pericardium 6 in relieving nausea. You might want to purchase acupressure wristbands to place over this point when you travel. When worn as directed, the nodules on the bands put pressure on points acupressure proponents say reduce nausea. The bands are often recommended by conventional physicians and alternative practitioners alike, and are sold in many pharmacies and travel-goods stores.

See the illustrations opposite for information on the location of Pericardium 6 and another point that may be helpful.

Aromatherapy
For relief of nausea, take 1 drop of the essential oil of peppermint *(Mentha piperita)* internally by mixing it with honey or a so-called carrier oil such as almond oil.

Ayurvedic Medicine
For adults, an Ayurvedic physician may prescribe the combined formula *Gasex* (two to three tablets chewed after meals); for children, *Bonnisan* (consult a practitioner for the proper dosage for your child's age). Another good remedy is an infusion or powder made from the bark and leaves of the neem tree.

Flower Remedies
The flower remedy Crab Apple is often recommended for motion sickness and other ailments

*M*otion Sickness

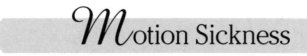

that cause nausea. Consult a naturopath or other practitioner familiar with flower remedies.

■ Herbal Therapy

Ginger *(Zingiber officinale)* is a favorite motion sickness remedy of naturopaths. The herb causes none of the side effects of antinausea drugs and can be drunk as a tea, eaten candied, or taken in capsule form (two capsules every four hours the day before and as needed during travel); it should be taken on an empty stomach.

■ Homeopathy

Homeopathic remedies sometimes come in kits that contain motion sickness remedies, which can be taken before and during travel as directed. One of the most effective is *Tabacum.*

■ Hydrotherapy

Placing an ice bag at the base of the skull and on the solar plexus for about 15 minutes can help relieve motion sickness. You might also try a hot compress on the abdomen, or bathing your feet in a pail of cold water (between 45°F and 55°F) for five to 10 minutes.

■ Massage

Properly administered, gentle massage to the chest and abdomen can help control motion sickness. First, however, you should make sure that your queasy stomach is not a symptom of a more serious problem, and you should discontinue the massage if your nausea increases.

Prevention

There are many strategies you can use to lower your vulnerability to motion sickness. In addition to the suggestions above, the following may help:

- Get plenty of fresh air. Open a car window, get on the ship's top deck, or open the overhead air vent in a plane.
- Keep your head as still as possible, close your eyes or focus on the horizon or another stationary object, and sit where motion is felt the least—in the front seat of the car, amidships or in a forward cabin of the ship, or over the wings of the plane. Avoid sitting facing backward on a bus, train, or plane. Don't read while in motion.
- Eat light meals of low-fat, starchy foods and avoid strong-smelling or -tasting foods.
- Don't drink alcohol or smoke.
- If nausea does set in, try eating olives or sucking on a lemon; these foods make your mouth dry and help diminish nausea. Soda crackers may help absorb excess saliva and acid in your stomach. If you feel too sick to eat, try drinking ginger ale (made from real ginger) or any carbonated beverage. ■

Acupressure

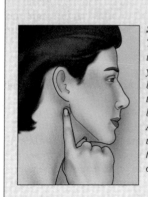

Small Intestine 17 • *To aid the ear's balancing mechanism, place your index fingers just below your earlobes in the indentations at the back of the jawbone. Apply light pressure while breathing deeply for one minute. Repeat one or two times.*

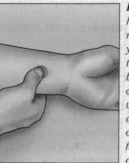

Pericardium 6 • *To help calm nerves and reduce nausea, place your thumb in the center of your inner wrist between the two forearm bones, two finger widths from the wrist crease. Press firmly for one minute, three to five times; then repeat on the other arm.*

$\mathcal{M}$uscle Cramps

Symptoms

Once you've experienced a muscle cramp, you'll probably recognize any future ones by the nature of the pain they cause. Common symptoms include:

- Sudden, painful spasm or tightening of a muscle, especially in the legs.

- Hardening of the affected muscle.

- In some cases, visible distortion or twitching of the muscle beneath the skin.

- In other cases, extremely severe cramps in the arms and legs, beginning without warning, and sometimes affecting the abdominal muscles as well. These symptoms are typical of heat cramps.

- Persistent cramping pains in lower abdominal muscles, which may occur along with back problems or during menstruation.

Call Your Doctor If

- you have frequent muscle cramps.

- your cramp lasts more than an hour and has not responded to your own treatment.

CAUTION

Cramping pain in your chest and arm muscles may indicate a heart problem. Call your doctor or get medical help immediately. If you suffer from circulatory problems, diabetes, heart disease, or deep varicose veins, or if you have had a stroke or been warned that you might be susceptible to one, avoid massage until you talk to your doctor.

F rom a stitch that grabs your side while you're running to a spasm in your calf awakening you in the dead of night, muscle cramps can be an all too common source of discomfort. Normally, a muscle at work contracts, then releases and lengthens when the movement is finished or when another muscle exerts force in the opposite direction. But sometimes a muscle contracts with great intensity and stays contracted, refusing to stretch out again; this is a muscle cramp.

Muscles contract or lengthen in response to electrical signals from nerves; minerals such as sodium, calcium, and magnesium, which surround and permeate muscle cells, play a key role in the transmission of these signals. Imbalances in these minerals—as well as in certain hormones, body fluids, and chemicals—or malfunctions in the nervous system itself can foul up the flow of electrical signals and cause a muscle to cramp.

Physical overexertion depletes fluids and minerals and can lead to cramping, particularly in people who work or exercise in conditions that overheat their bodies. If you are not careful to drink plenty of fluids, activities like working in the garden on a hot summer day can cause heat cramps. And if you do not take steps to alleviate them, heat cramps can progress to much more serious heatstroke and heat exhaustion.

Treatment Options

There are simple techniques for easing common, occasional muscle cramps (see Home Remedies, opposite), but if you suffer from frequent or severe cramps, see your doctor. Frequent cramps might indicate a more serious illness. And severe cramps in your chest, shoulders, or arms can be symptoms of a heart attack; call immediately for medical help.

Acupressure
If the cramp is in your calf, try applying pressure for two to three minutes at the lower end of the calf muscle bulge.

Aromatherapy
The essential oils of Roman chamomile, bay laurel (Laurus nobilis), and peppermint (Mentha piperita) may help relax tight muscles and soothe the pain of a muscle cramp; add a drop or two to a base oil and massage the muscle.

Muscle Cramps

Ayurvedic Medicine

An Ayurvedic physician may recommend massaging the affected area with oil of *shatavari* or applying a paste of ginger and turmeric.

Chinese Medicine

Chinese medicine offers a number of treatments for muscle cramps, including acupuncture and herbal medicine. Consult a practitioner.

Herbal Therapies

An infusion of ginkgo *(Ginkgo biloba)* may help improve circulation and relieve leg spasms. Pour a cup of boiling water onto 2 tsp of the dried herb and steep for 15 to 20 minutes; drink three times a day. An herbalist might prescribe Japanese quince *(Chaenomeles speciosa)* as an antispasmodic for cramps in the calves.

Homeopathy

Over-the-counter homeopathic preparations (in tablet form) of *Cuprum metallicum* (6c), sucked slowly, may relieve the spasm and ache.

Hydrotherapy

Use alternating hot and cold compresses: Soak one washcloth in hot water and another in ice water. Wring out the warm cloth, then place it over the affected area for three minutes. Wring out the second cloth and place it over the same area for 30 seconds. Repeat this alternating technique two more times. For severe cramping, do the procedure morning and evening; once a day for minor problems.

Or try a hot vinegar pack: Heat a pan of equal parts vinegar and water, then soak a towel in the mixture. Wring out the towel and apply it to the affected body area for five minutes. Remove the towel and apply a cold towel for five minutes. Cover with wool. Repeat these hot-cold applications three times, making sure to finish with cold.

Massage

A skilled practitioner can relieve cramping by applying massage directly to the affected area and using other cramp-releasing techniques. Massage is also useful for soothing the area and reducing tension once a cramp has released.

Nutrition and Diet

Nutritionists recommend taking vitamin E supplements (200 IU daily) to prevent night cramps. You may also find relief by increasing your intake of calcium. Good sources include milk, cheese, yogurt, dark green leafy vegetables, and canned fish. A 400-mg supplement taken before bed may help prevent night cramps.

Home Remedies

To relieve a typical cramp, you need to make the muscle stop contracting—by either stretching it or massaging it, or both. You can stretch a calf muscle simply by standing on your toes on the edge of a stair and slowly lowering your heels until you feel a good stretch without pain. For a greater stretch, stand facing a wall, put your hands or forearms against the wall, and—keeping your feet flat on the floor—slide backward until you are leaning against the wall from several feet away. For even more stretch, keep edging your feet backward.

Try this technique for massaging away a cramp: From a sitting position, stretch your heel down, pointing your toes up—toward your head. To give resistance, put your other foot against the top of the foot on the cramping side; then after the cramp releases, firmly squeeze your calf with your hand. Begin at the edges of the cramp and move in toward the center with gentle pressure. For an obstinate cramp, immerse the muscle in a hot bath, perhaps while stretching and massaging it. To treat heat cramps, drink plenty of cool water. This is also the best way to prevent heat cramps: Drink a cup of cool water before and after exercise, and every 15 minutes during exercise. If you use a sports beverage instead, drink one that is low in sugar (which can bring on stomach cramps). Dilute juices with 3 parts water.

Prevention

Practicing yoga regularly will greatly decrease the occurrence of leg cramps by stretching the muscles and increasing circulation. ∎

$\mathcal{N}$ausea

Symptoms

Symptoms of gastroenteritis, also called stomach flu or intestinal flu, include:

- Nausea and vomiting.
- Diarrhea.
- Abdominal cramps and pain.
- Fever.
- Weakness.

Any of a variety of mild to severe stomach symptoms may indicate gastritis. The most common are:

- Upper abdominal discomfort or pain.
- Nausea.
- Diarrhea.
- Loss of appetite.

Call Your Doctor If

- you have nausea with shortness of breath, chest pain, and sweating; these are signs of a heart attack.
- you experience nausea and severe headache, possibly with vomiting (these symptoms may worsen with exposure to bright light); you could have a migraine or meningitis.
- you have nausea accompanied by increased thirst and urination, dehydration, and possibly a fruity odor on your breath; you could have diabetes.
- you have severe nausea with pain starting in the upper abdomen and moving to the right shoulder blade; you may have gallstones.
- you have nausea that lasts one to two weeks, headache, malaise, and fatigue, perhaps accompanied by a sore throat, fever, and rash; possible disorders include mononucleosis, strep throat, and scarlet fever.

 *E*veryone has experienced the sick-to-your-stomach feeling of nausea at some point in life. Characterized by an urge to vomit, nausea is not itself an illness but rather a sign that things are not quite right in the digestive system or elsewhere in the body. The cause can be a relatively minor, temporary condition like motion sickness or anxiety, or as serious and life threatening as a heart attack or cancer of the stomach.

In many cases, nausea is brought on by a case of gastroenteritis, a general term that applies to many types of irritation and infection of the digestive tract. The most common cause of gastroenteritis is a virus that can spread quickly through an office, school, or day-care center. Food poisoning, bacteria, and parasites may also be the culprit, and sometimes drinking excessive amounts of alcohol can irritate your digestive tract enough to cause gastroenteritis.

Inflammation of the stomach lining, a condition known as gastritis, also commonly leads to nausea along with other symptoms such as vomiting, diarrhea, and general discomfort. Gastritis typically affects the elderly but can strike anyone at any age. It can be caused by certain medications, including aspirin, as well as by viral or bacterial infections.

Treatment Options

A number of alternative therapies can be extremely useful in treating nausea.

Acupressure

See the illustration opposite for an acupressure point that is particularly effective for relieving acute nausea and vomiting.

Aromatherapy

Essential oil of peppermint *(Mentha piperita)* can help calm the stomach and relieve a case of nausea. Take one drop internally by mixing it with honey or a so-called carrier oil such as almond oil.

Ayurvedic Medicine

A practitioner may recommend the combined formula *Gasex* for adults (two to three tablets chewed after meals) and *Bonnisan* for children (consult a practitioner for the dosage appropriate for your

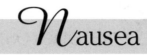 Nausea

child's age). Other appropriate remedies include a hot or cold infusion of the leaves of the neem tree, and a tea made from coriander seeds.

Chinese Medicine
After a thorough evaluation of your overall constitution, a practitioner of Chinese medicine can prescribe a course of treatment, which may include herbal therapy or possibly acupuncture, to harmonize the digestive organs.

Flower Remedy
The flower remedy Crab Apple is often recommended for ailments causing nausea. Consult a naturopath or other practitioner familiar with flower remedies.

Herbal Therapies
Meadowsweet *(Filipendula ulmaria)* can reduce nausea and stomach acidity: Pour 1 cup boiling water on 2 tsp dried meadowsweet and steep for 15 minutes; drink three times daily. Slippery elm *(Ulmus fulva)* may also help calm your digestive tract when the worst symptoms have passed: Mix 1 part powdered slippery elm with 8 parts water and bring to a boil; simmer for 15 minutes. Drink half a cup three times a day.

Chamomile *(Matricaria recutita)* tea can soothe the stomach: Steep 1 tsp of the herb in 1 cup of boiling water for 10 minutes. Licorice *(Glycyrrhiza glabra)* extract in capsule or liquid form may also help. Lemon balm *(Melissa officinalis)* is particularly good for digestive problems linked to anxiety. Ginger *(Zingiber officinale)* tea can help relieve nausea due to morning sickness, but check with your doctor before taking any herbal remedy.

Homeopathy
If symptoms are severe, take 12x dosages of one of the following homeopathic preparations every two hours until symptoms improve. If you do not feel any better after two or three doses, try another preparation:
- *Ipecac* for extreme nausea and vomiting.
- *Nux vomica* for symptoms caused by exhaustion, overeating, or drinking too much alcohol or coffee.

- *Bryonia* for nausea, a tender stomach, a dry mouth, and a sensation like a stone in your stomach.

Hydrotherapy
A cold footbath or ice bags at the base of the skull and on the solar plexus can help ease nausea. Another technique hydrotherapists often advise is placing a hot compress on the abdomen while applying a cold compress to the base of the skull.

Massage
Gentle massage of the chest and abdomen can provide relief from nausea. However, you must first make sure that your upset stomach is not a symptom of a more serious disorder. Massage is especially good for nausea related to anxiety and stress.

Nutrition and Diet
Limit or eliminate alcohol, caffeine, and carbonated drinks from your diet. When the worst symptoms have passed, eat more noncitrus fruit, cooked vegetables, and bland foods, and eat fewer refined carbohydrates such as white bread and white rice. Supplements of zinc and vitamin A may help heal the stomach lining after a bout with gastritis. ∎

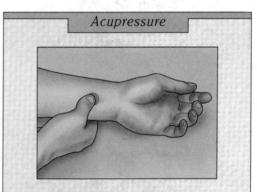

Acupressure

Pericardium 6 • *Pressing this point—between the two bones of the forearm, two finger widths from the center of the inner wrist crease—may help relieve nausea and stomach disorders. Press firmly for one minute, three to five times; then repeat on the other arm.*

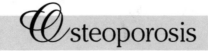steoporosis

Symptoms

Osteoporosis is usually asymptomatic until a fracture occurs.

- Backache.
- A gradual loss of height and an accompanying stooped posture.
- Fractures of the spine, wrists, or hips.
- Loss of bone in the jaw.

Call Your Doctor If

- you develop a backache or a sudden severe back pain, which can indicate a spinal compression fracture caused by osteoporosis.
- dental x-rays reveal a loss of bone in the jaw, which can be an early sign of osteoporosis.

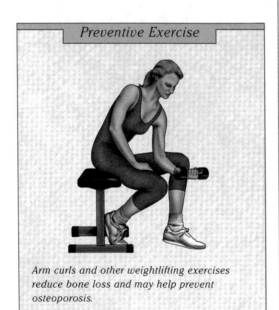

Preventive Exercise

Arm curls and other weightlifting exercises reduce bone loss and may help prevent osteoporosis.

O steoporosis, which means "porous bones," causes bones to gradually thin and weaken, leaving them susceptible to fractures. Although all bones are affected by the disease, those of the spine, hip, and wrist are most likely to break. In elderly people, hip fractures can be particularly dangerous, because the prolonged immobility required during healing often leads to blood clots or pneumonia. Women are more susceptible to osteoporosis, perhaps because their bones tend to be lighter and thinner, and because their bodies experience hormonal changes after menopause that appear to accelerate the loss of bone mass.

Treatment Options

Because osteoporosis is difficult to reverse, prevention is the key to treatment. To prevent the disease or slow its progression, many doctors suggest hormone replacement therapy to postmenopausal women. Many doctors recommend the treatment only for women at high risk of osteoporosis, because hormone replacement therapy has been associated with an increased risk of serious health problems, most notably uterine and breast cancers. Alternative medicine offers effective preventive measures that focus on building and retaining strong bones.

Exercise
Studies have shown that weight-bearing exercises—those that put stress on bones, such as running, walking, tennis, ballet, stair climbing, aerobics, and weightlifting—reduce bone loss and help prevent osteoporosis. To benefit from the exercise, you must do it at least three times per week for 30 to 45 minutes. Swimming and bicycle riding, although good cardiovascular exercises, do not appear to prevent osteoporosis because they do not put enough stress on bones.

Herbal Therapies
Herbs traditionally used to prevent osteoporosis include horsetail *(Equisetum arvense)*, alfalfa *(Medicago sativa)*, licorice *(Glycyrrhiza glabra)*, marsh mallow *(Althaea officinalis)*, and sourdock *(Rumex crispus)*. Take daily in tea or tincture form.

Chinese medicine herbalists may recommend

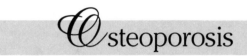

a general herbal formula used for graceful aging, *Liu Wei Di Huang Wan* (Six Flavor Pills); it is said to help nourish and strengthen the bones. Consult a practitioner for appropriate dosages.

■ Homeopathy

In addition to a calcium-rich diet and exercise, homeopaths recommend treatments they believe help the body absorb calcium. Remedies are likely to include *Calcarea carbonica*, *Calcarea phosphorica, Calcarea fluorica,* or *Silica*. Consult a homeopath for remedies and dosages.

■ Nutrition and Diet

To ensure that women get enough calcium to build and maintain strong bones, health experts recommend eating plenty of foods rich in calcium, such as nonfat milk, low-fat yogurt, broccoli, cauliflower, salmon, tofu, and leafy green vegetables. According to a panel convened by the National Institutes of Health, women who are still menstruating or who are postmenopausal but taking hormone replacement therapy should consume 1,000 mg of calcium each day. Postmenopausal women who are not being treated with estrogen should get 1,500 mg daily. (One glass of nonfat milk provides only 300 mg of calcium.)

Because most women take in through their diet only half or a third as much calcium as they need, some practitioners recommend calcium supplements to make up the difference. Calcium supplements are available in many forms, but chelated forms, such as calcium citrate and calcium gluconate, appear to be more effective at reducing bone loss. Avoid using dolomite or bone meal as calcium supplements or calcium carbonate supplements labeled "oyster shell," as they may contain lead and other toxic metals.

To help the body absorb calcium, some practitioners suggest taking vitamin D supplements (400 to 800 IU). Magnesium supplements (250 to 350 mg) or trace minerals are sometimes prescribed as well. CAUTION: Calcium supplements can inhibit the absorption of salicylates, tetracycline, and other medications. Check with your practitioner before beginning a supplementation program.

In addition to eating calcium-rich foods, you

should also avoid phosphorus-rich ones, which can promote bone loss. High-phosphorus foods include red meats, soft drinks, and those with phosphate food additives. Indeed, several studies have indicated that vegetarians tend to have denser bones later in life than meat eaters (other studies have shown no such difference).

To help keep estrogen levels from dropping precipitously after menopause and thus help prevent osteoporosis, some alternative practitioners advise postmenopausal women to consume more food containing plant estrogens, especially tofu, soybean milk, and other soy products.

Home Remedies

Here are two easy ways of increasing the amount of calcium in your diet:
- Add nonfat dry milk to everyday foods and beverages, including soups, stews, and casseroles. Each teaspoon of dry milk adds about 20 mg of calcium to your diet.
- Add a little vinegar to the water you use to make soup stock from bones. The vinegar will dissolve some of the calcium out of the bones, for a calcium-fortified soup. A pint can contain as much as 1,000 mg of calcium.

Prevention

- Eat foods rich in calcium, such as nonfat milk, low-fat yogurt, broccoli, salmon, tofu, sesame seeds, almonds, and leafy green vegetables.
- Eat foods that contain plant estrogens, especially tofu and other soy products.
- Avoid foods that can interfere with your body's absorption of calcium, such as red meats, soft drinks, and excessive amounts of alcohol and caffeine.
- Do weight-bearing exercises for 30 to 45 minutes at least three times a week.
- Do not smoke. Some studies have shown that women who smoke increase their risk of developing osteoporosis by 50 percent.
- Avoid antacids containing aluminum, as they can prevent calcium absorption by binding with phosphorus in the intestines. ■

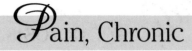

Pain, Chronic

Symptoms

Any pain that, despite treatment, lasts longer than six months is medically defined as chronic. The condition may include weakness, numbness, tingling, or other sensations along with sleeping difficulties, a lack of energy, and depression. Some common forms of chronic pain are:

- Continuing muscle pain, accompanied by cramping, soreness, swelling, and muscle spasms or stiffness.

- Lingering back pain, which may be sharp or aching, constant or intermittent, localized, radiating, or diffuse.

- Enduring joint pain, with tenderness and a sensation of heat in the affected area as well as radiating pain and a restricted range of motion.

Call Your Doctor If

- your pain continues for several weeks and doesn't respond to over-the-counter analgesics and rest; early care may keep acute pain from becoming chronic.

- your pain is unrelenting and unresponsive to prescription medications; your doctor may administer tests to rule out cancer or other possible causes.

- the symptoms of your chronic pain change abruptly. You may be at risk of complications, or you may have developed a different, unrelated problem.

T ens of millions of Americans suffer from chronic pain. It can be mild or excruciating, episodic or continuous, merely inconvenient or totally incapacitating. The emotional toll of chronic pain can become part of a vicious circle: Stress and anxiety may actually decrease the body's production of its natural painkillers. Because of the mind/body links associated with chronic pain, effective treatment may require addressing psychological as well as physical aspects of the condition.

Treatment Options

Many people suffering from chronic pain are able to gain some control over it on their own. But others may need professional help. For them, pain clinics—special care centers devoted exclusively to dealing with intractable pain—are often the answer.

Acupuncture

Acupuncture may be used to reduce swelling and inflammation associated with chronic pain. The treatment may include placing needles along the large intestine meridian, considered the most effective of pain-relieving channels. One theory holds that acupuncture works by stimulating the release of endorphins, the body's natural painkillers. Because this therapy is thought to have a cumulative effect, it is most beneficial if done on a regular basis. For the best results, consult an acupuncturist who has experience treating a wide range of types of chronic pain.

Aromatherapy

Mix together the following essential oils with a carrier oil such as sweet almond oil and massage the blend into your skin at the site of the pain: lavender *(Lavandula angustifolia)*, to reduce inflammation and relax muscles; eucalyptus globulus *(E. globulus)*, to bring down swelling and accelerate healing; ginger *(Zingiber officinale)*, to relieve pain and stiffness associated with arthritis and other types of degenerative joint disease.

Body Work

The Alexander technique reeducates you in the way you move to avoid adding unnecessary ten-

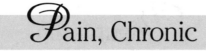 Pain, Chronic

sion to skeleton-supporting muscles, thus preventing neck and back problems. This therapy has been shown to be especially helpful for correcting poor posture that can cause backaches.

Exercise

Research has shown that regular exercise can diminish pain in the long run by improving muscle tone, strength, and flexibility. Exercise may also release endorphins. Some exercises are easier for certain chronic pain sufferers to perform than others; try swimming, biking, walking, or rowing.

Herbal Therapies

To help decrease inflammation and pain, herbalists recommend applying ginger *(Zingiber officinale)* packs, prepared by soaking a clean cloth in ginger tea, for 10 minutes, three to four times a day. Topically applied dilutions of wintergreen *(Gaultheria procumbens)* oil—which contains methyl salicylate, an ingredient similar to that found in aspirin—may have an analgesic effect. Geranium *(Pelargonium odoratissimum)* and white willow *(Salix alba)* bark are natural painkillers. Chamomile *(Matricaria recutita)* is an antispasmodic and anti-inflammatory agent. Consult an herbalist to determine the best treatment for your specific condition.

Homeopathy

Try *Rhus toxicodendron* for joint, back, and arthritic problems that feel worse when first rising in the morning and become better with warmth. Persistent, acute pain may be relieved by *Kali bichromicum*; however, a constitutional remedy is often needed to help relieve pain in the long run. Consult your homeopath for the correct constitutional remedy for you.

Massage

Massage therapy may provide temporary relief of muscle stiffness and spasms by reducing muscle tension, which can produce sudden, involuntary contractions that lead to more pain, which in turn leads to more spasms. Massage with ice packs may interrupt pain messages sent along nerve pathways, replacing those messages with signals about temperature and, in this way, providing relief.

Mind/Body Medicine

Visualization, or guided imagery, may be a worthwhile pain-controlling technique. Try the following exercise: Close your eyes and try to call up a visual image of the pain, giving it shape, color, size, and motion. Now try slowly altering this image, replacing it with a more harmonious, pleasing—and smaller—image. Don't expect this imaging technique to work right away; it takes practice.

Another approach is to keep a diary of your pain episodes and the causative and corrective factors surrounding them. Review your diary regularly to explore avenues of possible change. Strive to view pain as part of life, not all of it.

Electromyographic (EMG) biofeedback may alert you to the ways in which muscle tension is contributing to your pain and help you learn to control it.

Hypnotherapy and self-hypnosis may help you block or transform pain through refocusing techniques. One self-hypnosis strategy, known as glove anesthesia, involves putting yourself in a trance, placing a hand over the painful area, imagining that the hand is relaxed, heavy, and numb, and envisioning these sensations as replacing other, painful feelings in the affected area.

Relaxation techniques such as meditation have been shown to reduce stress-related pain when they are practiced regularly. Regular, gentle yoga practice can be helpful in relaxing muscles, thus decreasing pain and tension.

If you can't get your mind off the problems that may be producing stress, visualize two lists; in one column, list the problems in order of priority, and in the other, visualize potential solutions to them. Place an imaginary check mark by each one after you've found a solution for it, then put both lists out of your mind and try the relaxation exercise again.

Nutrition and Diet

For chronic back pain, a beneficial regimen may be 500 mg of vitamin C three times a day with meals, 800 mg daily of calcium taken with 400 mg of magnesium, and 400 IU daily of vitamin E. CAUTION: Be sure to check with your doctor or a nutritionist before taking large doses of vitamin supplements. ■

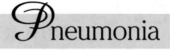
Pneumonia

Symptoms

- A combination of low fever and chills, muscle aches, fatigue, enlarged lymph nodes in the neck, chest pain, sore throat, and coughing are typical symptoms of viral pneumonia.

- High fever, cough with thick yellow-green sputum that may contain blood, shortness of breath, rapid breathing, sharp chest pain that is worse when you breathe deeply, abdominal pain, and severe fatigue are symptoms of bacterial pneumonia.

- Loss of appetite and weight, fever, coughing with sputum, perhaps following a period of unconsciousness, may indicate aspiration pneumonia.

- In children, labored and rapid breathing, sudden onset of fever, cough, wheezing, and bluish skin are general signs of pneumonia.

Call Your Doctor If

- your symptoms indicate you have any form of pneumonia. You need immediate medical treatment to recover and avoid complications.

- your sharp chest pain does not respond to prescribed treatment; you have increased shortness of breath; or your fingernails, toenails, or skin becomes dark or develops a bluish tinge after diagnosis. Your lungs are not getting enough oxygen and you need medical assistance.

- you cough up blood; you may need additional treatment for a worsening infection.

P *neumonia is the relatively common inflammation caused by various viral, bacterial, and fungal infections or by exposure of the lungs to certain chemicals. In response, the lungs become congested with fluids and cells that leak from the affected tissue. If the inflammation is limited to one lobe of one lung, it is classified as lobar pneumonia; inflammation spreading from the bronchi to other parts of one or both lungs is bronchopneumonia. If both lungs are inflamed, the condition is called double pneumonia.*

Treatment Options

If you are diagnosed as having pneumonia, various alternative therapies may help ease your symptoms and hasten your recovery.

Acupuncture

Acupuncture on the lung meridian may help your recovery from pneumonia by reducing cough and congestion, making you more comfortable, and improving your energy level. Consult a licensed practitioner for a complete evaluation so that the acupuncture treatments can be tailored to your specific condition.

Aromatherapy

Recovery from pneumonia may be helped if you add the essential oils of eucalyptus globulus (*E. globulus*), lavender (*Lavandula angustifolia*), tea tree (*Melaleuca alternifolia*), or pine to a warm bath or a vaporizer for steam inhalation.

Herbal Therapies

Since clearing the lungs of phlegm is an important part of the healing process, using traditional herbal expectorants to promote coughing can aid recovery. To make your own expectorant, combine 2 oz licorice (*Glycyrrhiza glabra*), 1 oz wild black cherry (*Prunus serotina*) bark, 1 oz coltsfoot (*Tussilago farfara*), ¾ tsp lobelia (*Lobelia inflata*), and 1 oz horehound (*Marrubium vulgare*). Simmer 1 tbsp of the mixture in 1 cup of water for five minutes; let the mixture steep for 10 minutes and strain it into a clean container. Adults should drink one cupful every two hours. Lobelia can be poisonous, so never use more than the recommended amount. Stop

*P*neumonia

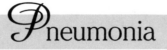

Evidence of Infection

Healthy lungs exchange carbon dioxide in the blood for oxygen through tiny air sacs called alveoli (inset, top). A pneumonic infection—whether it is caused by bacterial, viral, or chemical agents—makes tissue in the alveoli swell and fill with fluid (inset, bottom). Shallow, labored breathing brought on by an insufficient oxygen supply is often a symptom of pneumonia.

LUNGS

HEALTHY ALVEOLI

FLUID-FILLED ALVEOLI

using this mixture if you become nauseated, and never give it to children or pregnant women.

Homeopathy

Some recommended over-the-counter homeopathic remedies are *Aconite*, *Ferrum phosphoricum*, *Bryonia*, *Phosphorus*, and *Arsenicum album*; follow label directions. For lingering chest weakness after pneumonia, a homeopathic physician might prescribe *Stannum metallicum* or *Antimonium tartaricum*.

Massage

After the fever is gone, massage the chest and the upper back muscles to ease chest congestion. Adding a few drops of essential oil of eucalyptus globulus to the massage lotion may help to loosen and release phlegm.

Percussion massage techniques may help relieve congestion by dislodging phlegm so it can be coughed out. Use the cupping technique *(see the Gallery of Massage Techniques, page 128)* on the back and sides of the body over the area of the lungs. Allow the receiver to cough up phlegm as much as needed.

Nutrition and Diet

- Up to 1,000 mg of vitamin C an hour may offer substantial benefits in fighting pneumonia if started within two days of onset. Reduce the dosage if you develop diarrhea.
- From 25,000 to 50,000 IU of vitamin A daily, for not more than two weeks, may help support your respiratory and immune systems.
- Zinc supplements, up to 60 mg daily, may also help your immune system fight infection.
- 600 IU of vitamin E daily may help support damaged lung tissue.

Home Remedies

- A heating pad or hot-water bottle on the chest or back for 10 minutes several times a day can help relieve chest pain. Wrap the pad or bottle in a towel to prevent burning the skin.
- Try a traditional mustard poultice to loosen phlegm. Mix dry mustard with enough warm water to make a thick paste. Spread the paste on thin cotton or cheesecloth, fold, and place on your chest for several minutes, but don't overdo it: Mustard may cause blistering if it is left on bare skin too long.

Prevention

- Avoid smoking and exposure to tobacco smoke, which significantly damage the hair-like cilia that filter irritants from the lungs. Smoking weakens your ability to fight viral and bacterial agents that cause pneumonia. ■

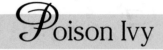

Poison Ivy

Symptoms

- Patches of red, itchy skin, usually followed by small blisters, which fill with a clear fluid and eventually break open.

- Severe cases can develop into swollen, extremely painful areas filled with fluid.

- The rash rarely appears on the soles of the feet or palms of the hands.

Call Your Doctor If

- your rash stays red and itchy for more than two weeks; you may have another type of contact dermatitis, eczema, or lupus.

- the rash is near your eyes or covers a large part of your body. You may need medical intervention.

- you have severe allergic complications, such as generalized swelling, headache, fever, or a secondary infection.

- you have been exposed to or inhale the smoke from burning poison ivy, poison oak, or poison sumac. The toxin is not killed by fire and can cause severe allergic reactions internally as well as externally.

Poison ivy, poison oak, and poison sumac cause a short-lived but extremely irritating allergic form of contact dermatitis. The rash generally develops within two days, peaks after five days, and starts to decline after a week or 10 days. While some people survive exposure without ill effects, complete immunity is unlikely; people who seem immune at one time and place may find themselves vulnerable in other situations.

The leaves, stems, and roots of these plants contain the resin urushiol, which even in minute amounts can trigger an inflammatory allergic reaction on exposed skin. Urushiol can be transferred by fingers or animal fur and can remain on clothing, shoes, and tools for several months. Scratching the rash does not spread the poison to other parts of the body, but it can prolong the discomfort and cause a secondary infection.

Treatment Options

You can treat a mild case yourself using conventional or alternative remedies. Conventional over-the-counter topical remedies contain antihistamines, benzocaine, or hydrocortisone, which relieve the symptoms of poison ivy. Various alternative therapies help relieve itching and swelling. In addition to topical remedies, vitamin C injections are also said to provide relief. If you have complications from a severe case, you may need to see a doctor. If your case is so severe that general illness develops, your doctor may recommend injections of prednisone or another corticosteroid drug.

Herbal Therapies

The leaves of jewelweed *(Impatiens pallida)*, which often grows near poison ivy, may neutralize urushiol if wiped over the skin immediately after contact. For relief from itching, try the following topical remedies:

- The leaves of the common plantain *(Plantago major)*. Make a poultice by mashing the leaves with a mortar and pestle. Apply the mashed leaves directly to the skin, then hold in place by covering with clean cotton or gauze strips.
- 1 tbsp salt in ½ cup water with enough cosmetic clay to make a paste; add 1 or 2 drops of oil of peppermint *(Mentha piperita)*.

$\mathcal{P}$oison Ivy

- Equal parts goldenseal *(Hydrastis canadensis)* root powder and green clay, available in health food stores.
- Osha *(Ligusticum porterii)* root tincture taken internally has an antihistamine effect that will reduce swelling. Take 20 drops of the tincture three times a day.

■ Homeopathy

Of all the over-the-counter homeopathic remedies available, *Rhus toxicodendron*—derived from the poison ivy plant itself—may be the most effective. Follow directions on the label.

Home Remedies

- Wash exposed skin with soap and water within 15 minutes of contact. If soap and water aren't at hand, but you're near a creek, wash with mud and water before waiting to wash again at home.
- Cover open blisters with sterile gauze to prevent infection.
- Make a paste with water and cornstarch, oatmeal, baking soda, or Epsom salt, and apply it to the rash. You can also use a paste made with baking soda and a few drops of witch hazel.
- Run hot water over the rash—as hot as you can stand it. The itching will intensify briefly, then abate, giving you several itch-free hours.

Prevention

The best way to deal with this poisonous threesome is to learn to recognize the plants, then steer clear of them. If you suspect contact with a poison plant, wash immediately and thoroughly with soap and water anything—your skin, clothes, shoes, tools—that might have picked up the plant's toxic resin. If you're going into poison-plant country, try one of the barrier lotions available from outdoor suppliers. The old folk tale about eating poison ivy leaves to make yourself immune is just that—a myth: Never eat the leaves or berries of wild plants. Many of them can cause dangerous reactions in humans. ■

Identifying Poison Plants

Poison ivy—with its shiny green, sometimes reddish, yellow, or orange leaves—shares with poison oak a characteristic three-leaf pattern. Poison sumac has paired, pointed leaves, sometimes with greenish white berries. The maps below show the distribution (in green) of each type.

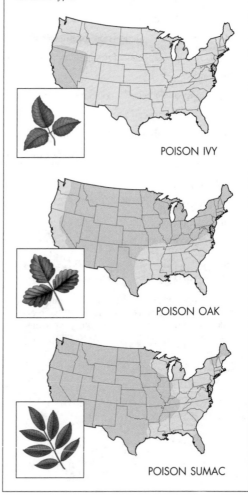

POISON IVY

POISON OAK

POISON SUMAC

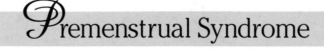
*P*remenstrual Syndrome

Symptoms

The symptoms of premenstrual syndrome recur during the same phase of the menstrual cycle, usually anywhere from seven to 10 days before your period begins. They may include any of the following:

- Bloating and fluid retention.

- Breast swelling and pain.

- Acne, cold sores, or susceptibility to herpes outbreaks.

- Weight gain of as much as five pounds (from retention of fluids).

- Headaches, backaches, and joint or muscle aches.

- Moodiness, anxiety, depression, or irritability.

- Food cravings, especially for sugary or salty foods.

- Insomnia.

- Drowsiness and fatigue, or conversely, extra energy.

- Hot flashes or nausea.

- Constipation, diarrhea, or urinary disorders.

A very small number of women with premenstrual syndrome may experience more intense symptoms:

- Fits of crying.

- Panic attacks.

- Suicidal thoughts.

- Aggressive or violent behavior.

Call Your Doctor If

- your symptoms are severe enough to interfere with your normal functions; your doctor may be able to offer treatments that will alleviate your symptoms.

*P*remenstrual syndrome—commonly known as PMS—is a physical condition characterized by a variety of symptoms that typically recur during a particular phase of the menstrual cycle. Practically every woman experiences at least one PMS symptom sometime in her life. Specific symptoms vary from woman to woman. Although some adolescents suffer from PMS, most women first develop the symptoms during their twenties.

Women most often affected by premenstrual syndrome are those who have experienced a major hormonal change, as may happen after childbirth, miscarriage, abortion, or tubal ligation. Women who stop birth-control pills may also notice an increase in PMS symptoms until their hormone balance returns.

Treatment Options

Remedies for PMS fall into two categories: hormonal treatments, prescribed by some conventional doctors, and nutritional and lifestyle changes, prescribed by both conventional and alternative practitioners. Hormones (usually estrogen or progesterone) are given in a variety of forms, including injection and vaginal or rectal suppositories. But because of the health risks associated with hormonal treatments, many women prefer to try alternative methods first. You may have to try several treatments, or a combination of them, before you find the right approach.

Aromatherapy
To relieve anxiety and irritability, add a few drops of lavender (*Lavandula angustifolia*) or German chamomile (*Matricaria recutita*) oil to a warm bath; juniper oil may also help. For breast tenderness, try adding 6 to 8 drops of geranium oil to a warm bath.

Herbal Therapies
Herbalists recommend a wide variety of herbs to help alleviate the many symptoms of PMS. Chaste tree (*Vitex agnus-castus*), for example, is sometimes prescribed because it is believed to help balance the body's hormones and relieve the anxiety and depression associated with PMS. Dandelion (*Taraxacum officinale*), whose leaves are thought to act as a powerful diuretic, is sometimes used to reduce

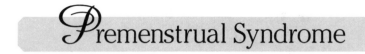 Premenstrual Syndrome

the bloating and breast swelling caused by premenstrual fluid retention.

For relief from PMS symptoms, Chinese herbalists sometimes recommend *Xiao Yao Wan* (Free and Easy Wanderer Pills). Consult a practitioner for the appropriate dosage.

■ Lifestyle

Studies have shown that regular exercise lessens PMS symptoms, perhaps by stimulating the release of endorphins and other brain chemicals that help relieve stress and lighten mood. Getting enough sleep is also important for the successful treatment of PMS. Lack of sleep can exacerbate fatigue, irritability, and other emotional symptoms. Experts recommend that people who have trouble getting enough rest stick to a regular sleep schedule.

■ Mind/Body Medicine

Various relaxation techniques, such as yoga and meditation, can be helpful in reducing the anxiety, irritability, and other emotional symptoms that sometimes occur premenstrually. The Cobra *(see page 38)* and Bow *(below, right)* yoga positions are particularly recommended for PMS.

■ Nutrition and Diet

Dietary changes have been shown to effectively reduce PMS symptoms in some women. Try reducing your intake of caffeine, sugar, salt, dairy products, and white flour, which studies have shown can aggravate your symptoms. Many women also find that eating six or more small meals throughout the day rather than three large ones reduces their symptoms, perhaps by keeping insulin levels more constant.

Some PMS symptoms, such as mood swings, fluid retention, bloatedness, breast tenderness, food cravings, and fatigue, have been linked to a deficiency of vitamin B_6 or magnesium. Nutritionists recommend supplements of these nutrients: 50 to 100 mg of vitamin B_6 daily, and 400 to 600 mg of magnesium daily, with a gradual increase if necessary. Supplements of calcium, zinc, copper, and vitamins A and E, as well as various amino acids and enzymes, are also sometimes prescribed. Consult an experienced nutritionist.

Some research has indicated that a dietary deficiency in fatty acids may contribute to PMS. Many women report that taking evening primrose *(Oenothera biennis)* oil, a substance that contains essential fatty acids, is effective. Your healthcare practitioner may recommend that you take one or two capsules (500 mg) up to three times a day throughout the month. Other dosage regimens are also recommended. Consult your healthcare practitioner.

Home Remedies

- Try to reduce stress and increase sleep during the week before your period.
- Exercise regularly.
- Try to manage your food cravings—particularly for chocolate; giving in to them may actually make your symptoms worse. Reach for fruit instead of sugary treats.
- As your period approaches, take long, warm baths to ease tension and stress.
- Use a hot-water bottle, a heating pad, or castor-oil packs to ease backaches and muscle aches associated with PMS.
- Abstain from alcohol before your period. It can aggravate PMS depression, headaches, and fatigue, and can trigger food cravings. ■

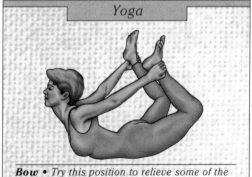

Yoga

Bow • *Try this position to relieve some of the symptoms of PMS. Lie on your stomach and grasp both ankles. While inhaling, squeeze your buttocks and slowly raise your head, chest, and thighs off the floor, pressing your ankles outward. Exhale and breathe slowly, then release.*

$\mathcal{P}$rostate Problems

Symptoms

For an enlarged prostate:

- Difficulties in urination, including a weak or intermittent stream, unusual frequency (especially at night), straining, dribbling, or inability to empty the bladder.

For acute prostatitis:

- Frequent, difficult urination.
- A burning sensation when urinating.
- Sudden fever, chills.
- Pain in the lower back and in the area just behind the scrotum.
- Blood in the urine.

For chronic prostatitis:

- Frequent, difficult urination.
- Pain in the pelvis and genital area.
- Pain upon ejaculation, blood in the semen, or sexual dysfunction.

For prostate cancer:

- A frequent need to urinate, especially at night; starting or stopping the urine stream may be difficult.
- A painful or burning sensation during urination or during ejaculation.
- Blood in urine or semen.

Call Your Doctor If

- your symptoms lead you to suspect an enlarged or infected prostate. If allowed to progress, prostate problems can lead to bladder stones, generalized infection, or kidney failure.
- your symptoms lead you to suspect you may have prostate cancer. However, in the early stages prostate cancer rarely causes symptoms. The American Cancer Society recommends that all men over the age of 50 have an annual PSA (prostate-specific antigen) test in order to detect early cancer.

T he prostate is a walnut-sized gland that surrounds the male urethra—the tube that transports urine from the bladder through the penis. Its primary function is to produce an essential portion of the seminal fluid that carries sperm; the prostate also controls the outward flow of urine from the bladder. Because of this dual role, signs of prostate trouble can include both urinary and sexual difficulties.

Prostate problems occur in two principal forms: enlargement of the prostate, or BPH (for benign prostatic hyperplasia), which appears to stem from age-related changes in hormonal balance; and prostatitis, a bacterial infection, which may be either sudden and severe (acute prostatitis) or milder but persistent or recurrent (chronic prostatitis). Prostatitis is often the result of a urinary tract or bladder infection that has spread into the prostate gland. A chronic infection may follow an acute one. An enlarged prostate can be a sign of prostate cancer.

Treatment Options

Various alternative remedies aim to relieve symptoms or shrink an enlarged prostate gland. If your symptoms are severe, you should see a physician.

Ayurvedic Medicine

A practitioner may prescribe herbal remedies and exercises to increase circulation and relieve congestion in the prostate.

Chinese Medicine

Prostatitis and urethritis are considered conditions of damp heat and would be treated accordingly by a practitioner.

Herbal Therapies

An extract of the berries of the saw palmetto (Serenoa repens), a scrubby tree of the American Southeast, is said to shrink an enlarged prostate and relieve symptoms. Other remedies include Asian ginseng (Panax ginseng), flower pollen, horsetail (Equisetum arvense), nettle (Urtica dioica), true unicorn root (Aletris farinosa), and the powdered bark of pygeum (Pygeum africanus), an evergreen tree.

For prostatitis, pipsissewa (Chimaphila umbellata) and horsetail are used to treat chronic infec-

$\mathcal{P}$rostate Problems

P

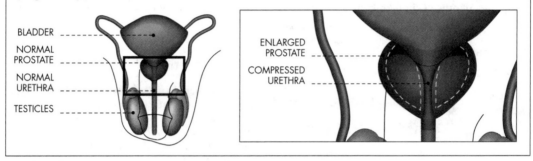

An Enlarged Prostate

The prostate, a walnut-sized gland in a man's lower abdomen, lies at the base of the bladder and surrounds a section of the urethra, a tube that carries urine and semen out of the body. As indicated below, enlargement of the prostate can put increasing pressure on the urethra, making urination progressively painful and difficult.

BLADDER
NORMAL PROSTATE
NORMAL URETHRA
TESTICLES

ENLARGED PROSTATE
COMPRESSED URETHRA

tion. Thuja *(Thuja occidentalis)* and pasqueflower *(Anemone pulsatilla)* are also suggested for inflammation of the prostate.

Homeopathy

Homeopathic practitioners may use various remedies to treat prostatic enlargement and prostatitis, among them *Berberis vulgaris* and *Staphysagria.*

Nutrition and Diet

Prostate enlargement may respond to nutritional therapies. Zinc, which is involved in many aspects of hormonal metabolism, is thought to promote prostate health and reduce inflammation; rich sources of zinc are oysters, wheat bran, whole oatmeal, pumpkinseeds, and sunflower seeds. Vitamins C and E may promote prostate health. The amino acids glycine, alanine, and glutamic acid are said to alleviate symptoms. The prostate may also benefit from large amounts of essential fatty acids, as found in flaxseed oil, walnut oil, sunflower oil, soybean oil, and evening primrose oil.

A recent study indicated that two to three servings a week of tomatoes—provided by food cooked in a tomato sauce, for example—may reduce the risk of prostate cancer, because of substances in the tomatoes called lycopenes.

Prevention

To prevent a recurrence of chronic prostatitis and promote prostate health:
- Take warm sitz baths.
- Drink water; dehydration stresses the gland.
- Avoid prolonged bicycle or horseback riding, or other exercises that irritate the area.
- Take supplements of zinc and vitamin C. ∎

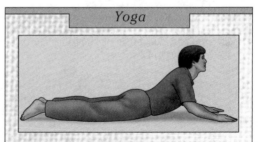

Yoga

Cobra • *For an enlarged prostate, place both forearms on the floor, elbows directly under your shoulders. Inhale and push your chest up while pressing your pelvis against the ground. Hold for 15 seconds, breathing deeply, then slowly relax.*

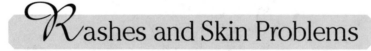

Rashes and Skin Problems

Symptoms

The general warning signs of skin cancer include:

- Any change in size, color, shape, or texture of a mole or other skin growth.

- An open or inflamed skin wound that won't heal.

Symptoms of other skin problems are varied:

- Dry, reddish, itchy skin indicates some type of dermatitis, or skin inflammation, of which there are many types.

- Deep pink, itchy, raised patches of skin with white scales, typically on the scalp, knees, elbows, and upper body, could be signs of psoriasis.

Call Your Doctor If

- an existing mole changes size, shape, color, or texture; you develop a very noticeable new mole as an adult; or a new skin growth or open sore does not heal or disappear in a few weeks. You may have skin cancer.

- a child's rash progresses rapidly from a simple red flush to small bumps, then becomes a crusted, pimplelike inflammation that's extremely itchy; the child probably has chickenpox.

- a child has a red rash that spreads from the face downward and is preceded by fever, cough, and inflamed nasal passages; these are symptoms of measles.

- you have painless ulcers on the genitals and perhaps in the mouth, followed by red, circular, non-itching lesions on the skin, especially the palms and soles; you may have syphilis.

T *he skin, largest of all human organs, is susceptible to a wide variety of disorders, ranging from short-lived and annoying rashes to painful, life-threatening skin cancer.*

Common Skin Problems

Among the most common skin problems is a broad range of ailments known as dermatitis, a term that means skin inflammation. One familiar type, contact dermatitis, typically causes the skin to develop a pink or red rash, which may or may not itch. Pinpointing the exact cause of contact dermatitis can be very difficult. The culprit can be a poisonous plant, such as poison ivy or poison oak, or one among any number of other possible irritants, including certain flowers, fruits, vegetables, herbs, detergents, soaps, antiperspirants, and cosmetics.

Atopic dermatitis—also known as eczema—causes the skin to itch, scale, swell, and sometimes blister. Eczema usually runs in families and is often associated with allergies, asthma, and stress. Seborrheic dermatitis is a condition that causes greasy, yellowish scaling on the scalp and other hairy areas, as well as on the face and genitals. In infants, the disorder is called cradle cap.

Another familiar malady of the skin is psoriasis. Unpredictable, intractable, and unsightly, this is one of the most baffling and persistent of all skin disorders. Psoriasis is characterized by skin cells that multiply up to 10 times faster than normal, typically on the knees, elbows, and scalp. As underlying cells reach the skin's surface and die, their sheer volume causes raised, white-scaled patches. A variety of factors, ranging from stress to a bacterial infection, can precipitate an episode of psoriasis. Many doctors believe external stress, such as that associated with a new job or the death of a loved one, triggers an inherited defect in skin-cell production. Psoriasis is not contagious, and most outbreaks are relatively benign. With treatment, symptoms generally subside within weeks.

Types of Skin Cancer

Skin cancers fall into two basic categories: melanoma and nonmelanoma. Melanoma is cancer of me-

Rashes and Skin Problems

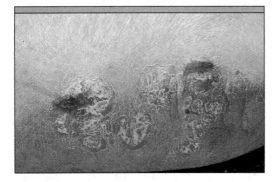

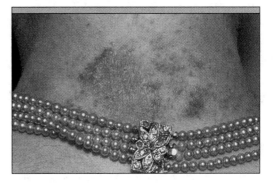

Psoriasis • *Usually occurring around the knees, elbows, and scalp, psoriasis is characterized by thick, silvery scales. There may be some itching but probably only a vague feeling of discomfort. Emotional stress and poor health can contribute to psoriasis; heredity is also a factor.*

Contact Dermatitis • *This rash results from contact with various substances, including certain plants, cosmetics, jewelry, medications, and detergents. Symptoms include small bumps or blisters that develop—over a period of weeks or months—into a rash that is usually very itchy.*

lanocytes, cells in the epidermis that produce a protective pigment called melanin; the disease affects about 1 in 10 skin cancer patients. It can start in heavily pigmented tissue, such as a mole or birthmark, as well as in normally pigmented skin. Melanoma usually appears first on the torso, although it can arise on the palm of the hand; on the sole of the foot; under a fingernail or toenail; in the mucous linings of the mouth, vagina, or anus; and even in the eye. Melanoma, which is associated with infrequent but excessive sunbathing that causes scorching sunburn, is an extremely virulent, life-threatening cancer. It is readily detectable and always curable if treated early, but it progresses faster than other types of skin cancer and tends to spread beyond the skin. Once this occurs, melanoma becomes very difficult to treat and cure.

The two most common skin cancers—basal cell carcinoma (BCC) and squamous cell carcinoma (SCC)—are nonmelanomas, which are rarely life threatening. They progress slowly, seldom spread beyond the skin, are detected easily, and are usually curable. BCC, which accounts for nearly 3 out of 4 skin cancers, is the slowest growing; SCC is somewhat more aggressive and more inclined to spread.

Every malignant skin tumor in time becomes visible on the skin's surface, making skin cancer the only type of cancer that is almost always detectable in its early, curable stages. Prompt treatment of skin cancer is equivalent to cure.

Treatment Options

Alternative therapies can be very useful in the treatment of many common skin problems. They can also help combat the pain, nausea, fatigue, and headaches that frequently accompany conventional treatment of advanced skin cancer. However, the only acceptable treatment for cancer is conventional medical care. If you think you have skin cancer, see a doctor without delay.

Aromatherapy

Essential oils of lavender *(Lavandula angustifolia)*, thyme *(Thymus vulgaris)*, jasmine, and German chamomile *(Matricaria recutita)* may help soothe allergy-related eczema when they are used to scent a room. Add a few drops of one of these oils to a bowl of hot water. (Do not apply the oils directly to the skin.)

Flower Remedy

Rescue Remedy is a cream that can be applied to a rash or other irritation as often as two or three

CONTINUED

*R*ashes and Skin Problems

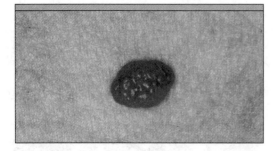

Mole • *Sometimes confused with melanoma, moles are benign growths that come in many shapes and sizes. They can develop at any age and on any part of the body. Most are dark and circular, and either smooth and flat or raised and wrinkled. If the color or size changes or if a mole starts to bleed, call your doctor.*

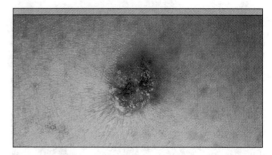

Basal Cell Carcinoma • *The most common type of skin cancer, basal cell carcinoma is a malignancy that grows slowly and rarely spreads to other organs. A small bump—typically in areas routinely exposed to the sun—develops a central crater that eventually erodes, crusts, and bleeds.*

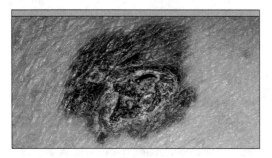

Melanoma • *The most serious form of skin cancer, melanoma may develop from an existing mole with an irregular border or in an area where there was no previous mole. The dark spot can become inflamed and change shape, color, size, and elevation. Call a doctor right away.*

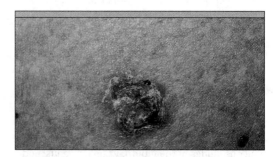

Squamous Cell Carcinoma • *Continual overexposure to the sun is the most frequent cause of this cancer. The tumor typically appears as a hard lump with a scaly, crusted surface. Growths usually develop on the lips, ears, hands, neck, and arms. This cancer can spread to internal organs.*

times a day. It can help reduce inflammation and speed the healing process.

▪ Herbal Therapies

Over the years, countless herbs have been used to treat skin ailments. Picking out what's right for your condition can be difficult, so seek help from a trained practitioner. The following are some substances herbalists consistently recommend.

Evidence suggests that evening primrose

(Oenothera biennis) oil may effectively soothe itching associated with dermatitis and psoriasis. Some doctors believe it's as effective as corticosteroid drugs with fewer side effects, although people with liver disease or high cholesterol should use it only under medical supervision; pregnant women should avoid evening primrose oil because it can affect hormone levels.

Burdock *(Arctium lappa)* root, which boosts the immune system and helps reduce inflamma-

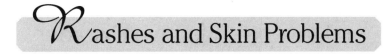

ℛashes and Skin Problems

tion, and dandelion *(Taraxacum officinale)* root may also help reduce symptoms of dermatitis and psoriasis. Simmer 1 tbsp of either of these dried herbs in a cup of boiling water for 10 minutes; strain and drink hot, up to 3 cups a day. You may also take up to 1½ tsp fluidextract of burdock or dandelion root daily.

▉ Homeopathy

For benign, short-term skin problems, an over-the-counter *Calendula* cream may soothe the inflammation. Taking *Rhus toxicodendron* (12x) three or four times a day may relieve the itching associated with a number of skin disorders, including contact dermatitis and chickenpox.

Don't try to choose homeopathic remedies on your own to treat a chronic, systemic condition such as psoriasis. Consult a qualified practitioner, who may recommend *Sulfur, Graphites, Lycopodium*, or *Arsenicum album*.

▉ Light Therapy

Psoriasis and certain chronic types of dermatitis often respond to light therapy (also called phototherapy), in which patients receive timed exposure to ultraviolet rays from an artificial light source. In nearly all cases, the skin clears considerably in a matter of weeks.

Despite its apparent effectiveness, light therapy has its drawbacks. At four to eight sittings a month, treatment can be time consuming and relatively expensive. Light therapy may cause premature aging of the skin and increase a person's risk of developing skin cancer. In some instances, the skin condition can recur within a year.

Some people try to avoid the doctor's office or the hospital by using a tanning salon as their source of UV radiation. They won't find the healing rays they seek, however. Because of concerns about the risks of skin cancer, tanning salons must filter out the type of UV rays used in light therapy. Even patients who own a sunlamp should seek help from a healthcare professional. Only a qualified practitioner can tell you how much UV radiation you can tolerate without risking long-term damage to the skin.

Some light therapists recommend the use of indigo light to treat allergic hives and insect bites.

▉ Nutrition and Diet

Fish oil high in EPA (eicosapentaenoic acid), from such fish as mackerel, herring, and salmon, may help reduce inflammation and itching. Because you would have to eat up to two pounds of fish a day to get enough EPA, try a 1,000-mg fish-oil capsule containing EPA four times a day; or try 1 tbsp cod-liver oil, also high in vitamin A, once a day; vitamin A plays a vital role in skin growth and maintenance.

Supplements of vitamin A (25,000 IU a day) and zinc (50 to 100 mg a day) may aid in skin healing, while vitamin E ointment or capsules (200 to 400 IU a day) can help relieve itching and dryness. Vitamin B complex containing vitamin B_5 and vitamin B_1 may also promote healthy skin: To help fight a case of psoriasis or dermatitis, the suggested dosage is 50 mg two or three times a day.

Home Remedies

- For dermatitis and mild forms of psoriasis, try mixing over-the-counter oatmeal or cornstarch preparations into a warm bath. Follow with application of a topical ointment (such as petroleum jelly or vegetable shortening) that helps the skin retain water and soothes inflammation. Take care not to stay in the bath too long: Lengthy immersion can strip the skin of essential oils.
- For scalp psoriasis, wash your hair with a coal-tar shampoo or with a mixture of cedarwood and juniper or lemon oils.

Prevention

If you are susceptible to skin cancer, take the following precautions whenever possible:
- Avoid intense sun exposure by staying out of it from late morning through early afternoon.
- Outside, wear a hat, long sleeves, trousers, and sunglasses that block UV radiation.
- Use a sunscreen with a sun protection factor of 15 or higher whenever you are outside.
- Consider taking a B-complex vitamin; B vitamins contain a compound called PABA, the active ingredient in many sunscreens. ▉

Seasonal Affective Disorder

Symptoms

Some or all of these symptoms are present during the fall and winter. Occasionally, seasonal affective disorder (SAD) occurs in summer, but with diminished rather than increased eating or sleeping symptoms.

- Depression, difficulty enjoying life, pessimism about the future.
- Loss of energy, inertia, apathy.
- Increased sleep, difficulty getting up in the morning.
- Impaired functioning: difficulty getting to work on time; tasks that are normally easy seem impossible.
- Increased appetite, weight gain.
- Carbohydrate cravings.
- Desire to avoid people.
- Irritability, crying spells.
- Decreased sex drive.
- Suicidal thoughts or feelings.

For children and adolescents:

- Feeling tired and irritable.
- Temper tantrums.
- Difficulty concentrating.
- Vague physical complaints.
- Marked cravings for junk food.

Call Your Doctor If

- you or your child suffers some of these symptoms with the onset of fall and winter and they seem to diminish or dissipate as spring and summer approach; your healthcare practitioner can help guide you to the most effective treatments for this condition.

 easonal affective disorder (SAD) is an extreme form of the "winter blues," bringing lethargy and curtailing normal functioning. It was only recently recognized as a specific disorder, but since 1982 much has been learned about it and how to treat it. People suffering from SAD undergo extreme seasonal differences in mood, as if they were split between a "summer person" and a "winter person."

Although a different kind of SAD can occur in the summer, its most common form begins gradually in late August or early September and continues until March or early April, when the symptoms begin to dissipate. Sufferers have been known to increase their sleep by as much as four hours a night and gain more than 20 pounds as they attempt to "hibernate" the winter away. Research suggests that SAD may affect 11 million people in the United States each year, and that an additional 25 million suffer a milder form that is indeed called the winter blues. Four times as many women suffer from SAD as men, and it tends to run in families.

The condition is thought to be caused by fluctuations in the brain chemical serotonin, which are triggered by inadequate amounts of outdoor light. Geographical location plays the largest role in determining a person's susceptibility to SAD; the nearer one lives to one of the poles, the greater the incidence.

Treatment Options

The most effective treatment for SAD is light therapy, sometimes combined with psychotherapy. However, a number of other alternative remedies have also proved helpful. For example, some healers believe that certain electrical emissions in the atmosphere—negative ions—improve a person's mood and health. In the last 30 years, scientists have developed small devices that emit negative ions into the atmosphere of a room. The negative ionizer seems particularly helpful for people with SAD (one study showed a 58 percent reduction of depression) and may be a good supplement to light therapy and medications.

Body Work

A number of people with seasonal affective disorder have found relief of their symptoms through Therapeutic Touch.

Seasonal Affective Disorder

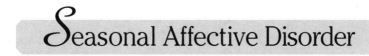

Chinese Medicine

SAD has been known to Chinese medicine for centuries and can be treated by acupuncture and Chinese herbs used in special combinations. Consult a practitioner for a course of treatment that is appropriate for your condition.

Energy Medicine

Polarity therapy, administered by a trained practitioner, can often be helpful in cases of SAD.

Flower Remedies

The Bach flower remedy Rescue Remedy is often recommended for patients with seasonal affective disorder and may be particularly beneficial when used in combination with other flower remedies. Consult a naturopath or other practitioner familiar with flower remedies.

Hydrotherapy

To help promote relaxation and ease depression, soak in a hot bath containing a few drops of lavender *(Lavandula angustifolia)* or German chamomile *(Matricaria recutita)* essential oil. Consult a naturopathic physician familiar with hydrotherapy for other appropriate remedies.

Light Therapy

Light therapy can be used in different ways and may employ different types of light boxes, light visors, and lamps. All are designed to bring extra light to the eyes. Check to be sure a light box filters out harmful ultraviolet light.

Light boxes that generate strong full-spectrum light are the most beneficial (strong fluorescent light may cause problems such as dizziness, headaches, and even depression). Place the box on a table or desk where you can do paperwork, read, or make phone calls, and sit before it for periods varying from 15 minutes to 1½ hours a day.

Other light sources include larger boxes that stand on the floor, visors with lights attached, and dawn simulators—lights programmed to turn on by your bed on winter mornings before dawn.

Light boxes can be bought for several hundred dollars at special stores. Experts warn against constructing your own light box because of possible damage from ultraviolet light.

Massage

Administered by a trained professional, massage may be a useful adjunct to other therapies. Try three or four massage sessions to see if it works; one session is not enough to judge.

Mind/Body Medicine

Tapping the power of the mind and spirit can be of immense value in overcoming SAD. Various forms of meditation help relax the body and focus concentration, and for many people the power of prayer can be formidable therapy. Others find relief through guided imagery, in which patients are trained to use their imagination as a way to influence certain physiological conditions. Exercise can also be very helpful; in particular, engaging in a regular program of yoga is said to be a powerful way to rebalance the endocrine system and thereby decrease the symptoms of SAD.

Nutrition and Diet

People with SAD are apt to overeat in the winter, with cravings for sweets and starches. One SAD expert urges patients to avoid snacking on foods rich in carbohydrates and, instead, balance carbohydrates with protein or restrict carbohydrate-rich food to a single balanced meal a day.

Home Remedies

- Take a walk at lunchtime when the sun is high. Be outdoors as often as you can.
- Exercise as much as you are able.
- Take winter vacations in places with long days.
- Increase the natural light in your home by trimming low-lying branches near the house and hedges around windows.
- Paint your walls with lighter colors.
- Keep warm and enjoy the fun aspects of winter—such as wood fires, books, music. ■

Sinusitis

Symptoms

- Feeling of fullness in the face.
- Pressure behind the eyes.
- Nasal obstruction, difficulty breathing through the nose.
- Postnasal drip.
- Foul smell in the nose.
- Fever (possibly).
- Toothache (possibly).

Call Your Doctor If

- sinusitis develops into an inflammation around the eye (orbital cellulitis), which could cause damage to the eye and facial nerves.
- the condition does not improve within seven days; you may need a prescription for antibiotics.
- sinusitis recurs more than three times in a year, and periods between bouts grow shorter; you may have a chronic infection that could become serious.

Sinusitis is an infection or inflammation of the sinuses, the air-filled pockets in the bones of the face. One of the most common healthcare complaints in the U.S., sinusitis occurs when the mucus-producing linings of the sinuses become inflamed. By far the most frequent cause is blockage of the tiny drainage openings called ostia, perhaps as a result of an upper respiratory tract viral infection. Once these openings are clogged, foreign material can't get out, and invading bacteria cause the sinus walls to swell and fill with pus.

Treatment Options

Many alternative therapies attempt to relieve the pain of sinusitis and open the sinuses for drainage. Others aim to fight infection by boosting the immune system. If the sinuses are infected with bacteria, you may need antibiotics to kill the disease organisms before they cause further damage or spread to other sinuses.

Acupuncture

Acupuncture has been shown to be effective in the treatment of sinusitis. An acupuncturist may apply medium stimulation to various ear points—adrenal, forehead, internal nose, lung, and near the sinuses—to help drain the sinuses. Points on the stomach, bladder, and large intestine meridians can also help; consult a licensed practitioner.

Aromatherapy

Inhalants of eucalyptus globulus (E. globulus), pine, or thyme (Thymus vulgaris) may help break up your clogged sinuses. You may also alleviate the symptoms by holding menthol or eucalyptus packs over your sinuses.

Herbal Therapies

Bromelain tablets have been shown in controlled studies to reduce inflammation, nasal discharge, headache, and breathing difficulties. You can boost your immune system with echinacea (Echinacea spp.), goldenseal (Hydrastis canadensis), or garlic (Allium sativum), preferably raw. Breathing the steam of clove (Syzygium aromaticum) tea or ginger (Zingiber officinale) tea also provides some relief. To combat excessive mucus production, herbalists

$\mathcal{S}$inusitis

suggest elder *(Sambucus nigra)* flower, eyebright *(Euphrasia officinalis)*, marsh mallow *(Althaea officinalis)*, or goldenrod *(Solidago virgaurea)*.

The exact makeup of a prescribed Chinese herbal mixture depends on whether the sinusitis is "hot" (acute or infectious) or "cold" (chronic or allergic). Either way, the preparation may include the Chinese herb ephedra *(Ephedra sinica)*, a decongestant. (WARNING: Do not use ephedra if you have hypertension or heart disease.) A number of other Chinese herbs, among them honeysuckle *(Lonicera japonica)*, fritillary bulb *(Fritillaria cirrhosa)*, tangerine peel *(Citrus reticulata)*, xanthium fruit *(Xanthium sibiricum)*, and magnolia flower *(Magnolia liliflora)*, can also help relieve sinusitis symptoms.

■ Homeopathy

For acute sinusitis with thick, stringy mucus and pain in the cheeks or the bridge of the nose, use *Kali bichromicum* (30c) once or twice a day. For sinusitis with intense facial pain, alternating chills and sweat, and yellow-green discharge from the nose and mouth, use *Mercurius vivus* (30c) twice a day. For acute sinusitis with a clear, thin discharge, sneezing, headache, and a stopped-up nose at night, use *Nux vomica* (30c) twice a day. For sinusitis with light yellow or green nasal discharge accompanied by low spirits and lack of thirst, use *Pulsatilla* (30c) twice a day. If symptoms linger for more than two days, seek the advice of a professional homeopath.

■ Nutrition and Diet

A good, healthful diet including fruits and raw green leafy vegetables can help stimulate secretions and break up sinusitis. Nutritionists also suggest the following supplements to the diet: vitamin C, 500 mg every two hours; bioflavonoids, 1 gram per day; beta carotene (vitamin A), 25,000 IU per day; and zinc lozenges (consult a nutritionist for dosages). Stay away from foods that you suspect may trigger an allergic reaction.

Home Remedies

■ Inhale steam from a vaporizer, a humidifier, a mixture of hot water and vinegar, or even a cup of tea or coffee. Steam is one of the best remedies for unclogging sinuses.
■ Use warm compresses on your nose to help open your sinuses.
■ Drink plenty of liquids.

Prevention

It's difficult to prevent sinusitis, but you can reduce your chances of having your sinuses become infected. First, avoid allergenic substances, which for some people include the dust in their beds and certain foods, such as dairy products and wheat. Whenever possible, avoid cigarette smoke. Note: People with diabetes, cystic fibrosis, and certain other diseases may be prone to sinusitis. ■

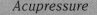

Acupressure

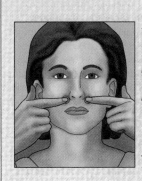

Large Intestine 20 •
This point may help relieve the pain, congestion, and swelling of sinusitis. Gently press the points on either side of your nose; apply pressure upward, underneath your cheekbones. Breathe deeply and hold for one minute.

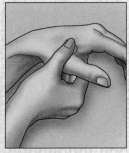

Large Intestine 4 •
To ease headache pain and congestion, press your right thumb into the webbing between the thumb and index finger of your left hand. Hold for one minute, then repeat on the other hand. (Do not use if you are pregnant.)

$\mathcal{S}$ore Throat

Symptoms

The classic symptoms of a sore throat include a burning sensation or "scratchiness" in the back of the throat; pain, especially when swallowing; and, perhaps, tenderness along the neck. These symptoms may be accompanied by:

- Sneezing and coughing.
- Hoarseness.
- Runny nose.
- Mild fever.
- General fatigue.

Call Your Doctor If

- you also have a fever higher than 101°F without other cold symptoms; this may indicate a case of strep throat, which needs treatment.
- you also have flulike symptoms that don't get better after a few days; this may indicate infectious mononucleosis.
- any hoarseness lasts longer than two weeks; this could be a sign of throat cancer or oral cancer.
- your sore throat is accompanied by drooling, or you experience difficulty swallowing or breathing; this may indicate an inflamed epiglottis, the structure that overhangs the opening to the larynx, or an abscess in the back of the throat; these two uncommon conditions require medical attention.

S ore throat is one of the most common health complaints, particularly during the colder months, when respiratory diseases are at their peak. Typically the raw, scratchy, burning feeling at the back of your throat is the first sign that a cold or the flu is on the way. But a sore throat can also presage more serious conditions, so you should watch how it develops and call a doctor if it seems to be out of the ordinary.

Treatment Options

Most alternative therapies for sore throat are geared toward symptom relief, although some address the cause. A sore throat usually goes away on its own. However, if the pain persists or worsens after a few days, you should see your doctor.

Aromatherapy

To increase blood circulation and improve fluid drainage in sore areas, massage your throat and chest with a lotion made with 2 drops each of eucalyptus globulus (E. globulus) and cypress in 2 tsp of a carrier oil such as vegetable or almond oil.

Herbal Therapies

At the first sign of soreness, take three raw cloves of garlic (Allium sativum) a day. (Garlic is a natural antibiotic and antiseptic.) If garlic smell becomes a problem, try four garlic oil capsules instead. Teas made from either goldenseal (Hydrastis canadensis) or echinacea (Echinacea spp.) may also be effective. One of the best herbal treatments uses ginger (Zingiber officinale), which is noted for its anti-inflammatory properties. Simmer 2 tsp chopped fresh ginger in water for 20 minutes; breathe in the steam from this tea for five minutes and repeat two or three times a day.

A traditional Native American treatment is drinking a tea made from the inner bark of the slippery elm (Ulmus fulva). Put 2 tsp powdered bark in 1 cup water. Bring to a boil and simmer for 10 to 15 minutes.

Homeopathy

Homeopaths prescribe several remedies for sore throats. Consult a homeopathic practitioner or try those listed here:

$\mathcal{S}$ore Throat

- If the pain comes on suddenly and is accompanied by great thirst and hoarseness, try *Aconite* (6c) three times a day.
- If the pain comes on suddenly and is accompanied by fever, headache, and restlessness, use *Belladonna* (6c) three times a day.
- If your sore throat has come on gradually and is accompanied by fatigue, try *Ferrum phosphoricum* (6c) three times a day.
- If the back of your throat is red and swollen and the pain is relieved by cold water or ice, try *Apis* (6c) three times a day.
- If your sore throat is accompanied by flulike symptoms, extreme sluggishness, and weakness, use *Gelsemium* (6c) three times a day.

■ Nutrition and Diet

At the first sign of soreness, take 500 to 6,000 mg of vitamin C daily to help fight the cold or other viral infection causing it. CAUTION: Unless your body is accustomed to megadoses of vitamin C, it cannot absorb more than about 1,000 mg every two hours; the excess will be passed off in your urine or, in some cases, result in diarrhea.

Home Remedies

- Get plenty of rest and drink a lot of fluids.
- Suck on a zinc lozenge (consult a nutritionist for dosages). Zinc can relieve sore throats and other cold symptoms but may cause nausea if taken on an empty stomach.
- To help relieve the pain, apply a warm heating pad or compress to your throat. You can also try a warm chamomile poultice: Mix 1 tbsp dried chamomile *(Matricaria recutita)* into 1 or 2 cups boiling water; steep for five minutes, then strain. Soak a clean cloth or towel in the tea, wring it out, then apply to your throat. Remove the cloth when it becomes cold. Repeat as often as necessary.
- Try steam inhalations to ease the pain. Run very hot water in a sink. With a towel draped over your head to trap the steam, lean over the sink while the water is running. Breathe deeply through your mouth and nose for five to 10 minutes. Repeat several times a day. ■

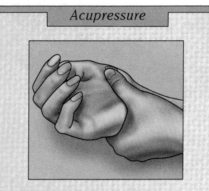

Acupressure

Lung 10 • *To help relieve the discomfort of a sore and swollen throat, try pressing on this point. Using your left thumb, apply pressure to the center of the pad at the base of your right thumb. Hold for one minute and repeat on the other hand.*

OF SPECIAL INTEREST

Homemade Gargles

To wash away mucus and irritants and bring relief from the pain of a sore throat, try any of the following gargles:

- *Salt water: Mix ½ tsp salt in 8 oz warm water.*
- *Sage: Put 1 to 2 tsp dried leaves in 1 cup boiling water; steep for 10 minutes, then strain and cool until lukewarm.*
- *Lemon: Mix the juice of one lemon in 8 oz warm water.*
- *Horseradish: Mix 1 tbsp pure horseradish, 1 tsp honey, and 1 tsp ground cloves in 8 oz warm water.*
- *Raspberry: Put 1 to 2 tsp raspberry leaf in 1 cup boiling water; steep for 10 minutes, then strain and cool until lukewarm.*
- *Cayenne pepper: Mix the juice of half a lemon, 1 tbsp salt, and ¼ tsp cayenne pepper (or more if you can tolerate it) in ½ cup warm water. The cayenne pepper temporarily reduces the amount of pain-causing chemicals produced by nerve endings in the throat.*

Stomach Ulcers

Symptoms

- Burning upper abdominal pain, particularly between meals, early in the morning, or after drinking orange juice, coffee, or alcohol, or taking aspirin; discomfort is usually relieved after taking antacids or eating a meal.

- Tarry, black, or bloody stools.

Call Your Doctor If

- you have been diagnosed with a stomach ulcer and begin experiencing symptoms of anemia, such as fatigue and a pallid complexion. Your ulcer may be bleeding.

- you have symptoms of a stomach ulcer and develop severe back pain. Your ulcer may be perforating the stomach wall. Call your doctor now.

- you have symptoms of a stomach ulcer and vomit blood or material that looks like coffee grounds, or you pass dark red, bloody, or black stools, or stools that resemble currant jelly. These symptoms indicate internal bleeding; call 911 or your emergency number now.

- you have an ulcer and become cold and clammy, and feel faint or actually do faint. These are symptoms of shock, usually resulting from massive blood loss; get emergency medical treatment.

 bout 1 out of 10 Americans will suffer from the burning, gnawing abdominal pain of an ulcer sometime in life. Stomach, or peptic, ulcers are holes or breaks in the protective lining of the stomach, the esophagus, or the duodenum, which is the upper part of the small intestine. The most common type are duodenal ulcers; the second most common are gastric ulcers, which develop in the stomach, followed by the comparatively rare esophageal ulcers, which are typically a result of alcohol abuse.

Although stress and diet have long been thought to cause ulcers, research conducted since the mid-1980s has persuasively demonstrated that the primary culprit in most ulcers is a bacterial infection; the bacterium Helicobacter pylori is present in 92 percent of duodenal ulcer cases and 73 percent of gastric ulcers.

Treatment Options

An ulcer should always be monitored by your doctor. When a bacterial infection has been diagnosed as the cause, the best treatment is with antibiotics, which can permanently cure the ulcer. Many people also use over-the-counter antacids for symptom relief. There are, however, a variety of alternative treatments that can aid in relieving pain and in healing ulcers.

Acupuncture
Acupuncture targeting the points associated with stress, anxiety, and stomach/gastrointestinal disorders may help with the treatment of peptic ulcers. Consult a licensed acupuncturist.

Herbal Therapy
Licorice *(Glycyrrhiza glabra)*, which stimulates mucus secretion by the stomach, is frequently used in herbal treatments of ulcers. Herbalists and naturopathic physicians typically employ a special preparation of licorice rather than the tincture or tea form; consult an herbal practitioner.

Mind/Body Medicine
Biofeedback, meditation, and other relaxation techniques can help you learn how to deal effectively with stress, which increases stomach acid production and irritates ulcers.

Stomach Ulcers

A Hole in the Stomach

A peptic ulcer is a break in the protective lining of the esophagus, the stomach, or the duodenum. Duodenal and gastric ulcers (inset) are the two commonest forms. Their typical symptoms are recurring pain in the upper abdomen and a bloated feeling after eating.

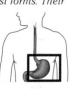

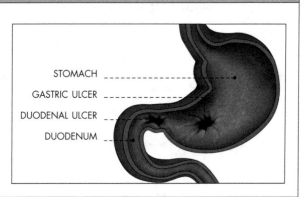

STOMACH

GASTRIC ULCER

DUODENAL ULCER

DUODENUM

Nutrition and Diet

Some nutritionists recommend supplementing your intake of vitamins A and E as well as zinc, which increase the production of mucin, a substance your body secretes to protect the stomach lining. Another suggestion may include drinking about a quart of cabbage juice daily; its high content of glutamine is thought to expedite the growth of mucin-producing cells.

Home Remedies

- Cut down on milk. Although it may feel as though milk's coating properties are soothing your ulcer, milk actually stimulates stomach acid secretion, irritating the ulcer.
- Pick appropriate antacids. Like milk, calcium-containing antacids can stimulate stomach acid secretion. Experiments suggest that bismuth, an ingredient in some over-the-counter stomach medications, may help destroy the bacterium that causes some peptic ulcers.
- Be cautious when choosing over-the-counter pain relievers. Aspirin and nonsteroidal anti-inflammatory drugs (NSAIDs), such as ibuprofen, can cause ulcers and prevent an existing ulcer from healing. Your best choice may be acetaminophen, which does not cause or promote stomach ulcers.
- Learn how to deal with stress. While there is no evidence that stress causes ulcers, it can

exacerbate existing ones. Practicing relaxation techniques can help alleviate stress.

Prevention

- Avoid foods and beverages such as caffeinated drinks that irritate your stomach. Use common sense: If it upsets your stomach, avoid it. Spicy and fatty foods are common irritants.
- Eat foods with high fiber content. Fiber is thought to enhance mucin secretion. ∎

OF SPECIAL INTEREST

Can You Catch an Ulcer?

In 1982, two Australian doctors determined that the bacterium Helicobacter pylori played a significant role in the development of peptic ulcers, and further studies have shown antibiotics to be effective in treating ulcers caused by the bacterium. Does this mean that ulcers are contagious? The answer is murky. Not everyone infected with the bacterium develops an ulcer, and certainly other factors—such as heredity and excessive use of aspirin, tobacco, and alcohol—increase the chances of getting one. Still, research has shown that infected children are more likely to transmit the bacterium than adults are.

Stress

Symptoms

- Physical symptoms may include headache, fatigue, insomnia, digestive changes, neck pain or backache, loss of appetite, or overeating.

- Psychological symptoms may include tension or anxiety, anger, reclusiveness, pessimism, resentment, increased irritability, feelings of cynicism, and inability to concentrate or perform at usual levels.

Call Your Doctor If

- you have prolonged or acute symptoms. Excessive stress puts you at risk of other serious disorders, including immune problems, digestive disorders, diabetes, asthma, high blood pressure, migraine headaches, and possibly cancer.

- you have symptoms of stress and any of the following: unusual patterns of sleep, appetite, and moods; physical movement that is unusually agitated or abnormally slow. You may have clinical depression.

Stress is the reaction of our bodies and minds to something that upsets their normal balance. The human response to stressful events is an ancient one, dating back to a time when life was a constant struggle for survival. A good example of stress in action is the way you react when you are frightened or threatened. But not all stressful events are so sudden or so obvious as the threat of bodily harm. Stress occurs when there is an imbalance between the demands of life and our ability to cope with them. Any challenge that overwhelms us—a serious illness, the death of a family member, the loss of a job or a lover—can be stressful to the point of physical and psychological dysfunction.

Treatment Options

Some treatments once considered alternative are now widely used in the medical community—particularly those designed to promote physical and mental relaxation.

Aromatherapy
Essential oil of lavender *(Lavandula angustifolia)* can help reduce stress: Try 5 or 6 drops in a bath, or put 2 or 3 drops on a handkerchief and inhale from time to time. Other oils to try include Roman chamomile *(Anthemis nobilis),* marjoram *(Origanum majorana),* lemon-scented eucalyptus *(Eucalyptus citriodora),* and lemon balm *(Melissa officinalis).*

Ayurvedic Medicine
Two combined formulas, *Geriforte* and *Mentat,* may help reduce stress. The following remedies may also be useful: a milk decoction or powder of the root of winter cherry; a decoction or powder of the fruit of emblic myrobalan; or an infusion, powder, or pill of gotu kola.

Body Work
The Alexander technique focuses on ways to eliminate stress-causing muscle tension and promote a restful breathing pattern.

Exercise
Vigorous aerobic exercise can reduce the level of pulse-quickening hormones released during stress and stimulate a sense of well-being. Even a walk

Yoga

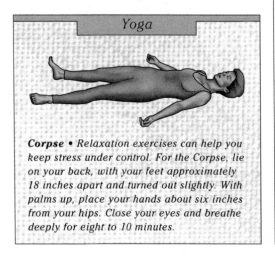

**Corpse • ** *Relaxation exercises can help you keep stress under control. For the Corpse, lie on your back, with your feet approximately 18 inches apart and turned out slightly. With palms up, place your hands about six inches from your hips. Close your eyes and breathe deeply for eight to 10 minutes.*

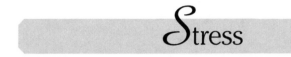

Stress

around the block can help reduce anxiety. Try to schedule the exercise of your choice for 30 minutes at least three times a week.

Stretching exercises can relax tense upper-body muscles that accompany stress and affect breathing. Rotate your shoulders up, back, and then down. Inhale as the shoulders go back; exhale as they go down. Do the exercise four or five times, inhale deeply, and exhale. Repeat the cycle.

Flower Remedy
The Bach flower Rescue Remedy may help reduce stress. Consult a naturopath or other practitioner familiar with flower remedies.

Herbal Therapies
A traditional response to stress is to drink a cup of hot tea. Some herbalists suggest chamomile *(Matricaria recutita)*, passionflower *(Passiflora incarnata)*, valerian *(Valeriana officinalis)*, or American ginseng *(Panax quinquefolius)* tea.

Hydrotherapy
Try a warm bath containing 1 drop of the essential oils of lavender *(Lavandula angustifolia)*, jasmine, or German chamomile *(Matricaria recutita)*.

Massage
By relaxing tense muscles and helping circulation, massage helps the mind relax. Between treatments, massage your temples, neck, shoulders, and face.

Mind/Body Medicine
Meditation brings relaxation and increased awareness. When you feel stressed, think affirmations such as "I can face this calmly. I control my own life." Or try visualization, or guided imagery, exercises. Visualizing a pleasant situation can bring physical as well as emotional benefits; combine a visualization session with soothing music. Many excellent teachers, books, and tapes are available to help you learn the technique.

Nutrition and Diet
How well you handle stress can be affected by your diet. Because it is easy to neglect nutrition when you are under stress, make an extra effort to eat a balanced diet—plenty of vegetables and fruit, as well as foods high in complex carbohydrates, moderate in protein, and low in fat. Avoid or reduce caffeine consumption: Excessive caffeine has been shown to increase anxiety.

Sound Therapy
A number of sound-therapy techniques can help reduce stress.

Home Remedies

There are many simple, inexpensive ways to manage stress on your own. For many people, a good way to start is by cutting out artificial stress relievers such as alcohol, which can mask symptoms and may become addictive. Try exercise instead. Take walks. Breathe deeply.

In times of stress, social support is crucial. People with close personal relationships are the most likely to recover from serious illness or injury, and stress is no different. The ability to form relationships with people—or pets, for that matter—can be a key to good health.

Prevention

While we can't—and perhaps shouldn't try to—change our personality or avoid stressful situations, we can learn to cope with them. Try the following:
- Cultivate outside interests and plan occasional diversions to break routine habits.
- Set up a regular sleeping schedule and get plenty of rest—without sleeping pills.
- Avoid the learned behaviors of hurry and worry, which can upset your sleeping, eating, and other schedules. Take time to enjoy your life.
- Make a list of things that trouble you. Ask yourself: What's the worst that can happen? Have I done what I can to prepare myself? Is this problem really worth worrying about?
- When you're facing a stressful situation, remember a bit of folk wisdom: Count to 10 and take a deep breath before saying or doing anything. A deliberate pause can be an instant tranquilizer. ∎

Sty

Symptoms

- Sty: a red, hot, tender, uncomfortable, and sometimes painful swelling near the edge of the eyelid. *(See the photograph opposite, below.)*

- Chalazion: a relatively painless, smooth, round bump within a fat gland of the eyelid.

Call Your Doctor If

- either type of swelling does not subside within a few weeks.

- the swelling interferes with your vision.

- you have pain in the eye.

- you have recurrent sties. A sty can be a symptom of other ailments such as diabetes and chronic skin problems.

A sty is a pimple or abscess on the upper or lower edge of the eyelid that signals an infected eyelid gland. Although sties are usually on the outside of the lid, they can also occur on the underside.

An external sty starts as a pimple next to an eyelash. It turns into a red, painful swelling that usually lasts several days before it bursts and then heals. Most external sties are short lived.

An internal sty (on the underside of the lid) also causes a red, painful swelling, but its location prevents the pus from appearing on the eyelid. The sty may disappear completely once the infection is past, or it may leave a small fluid-filled cyst or nodule that can persist and may have to be cut open.

A chalazion is also a sign of an infected eyelid gland, but unlike a sty, it is a firm, round, smooth, painless bump located usually some distance from the edge of the lid.

Sties and chalazions are usually harmless and rarely affect your eye or sight. They can occur at any age and tend to recur elsewhere on the lid.

Treatment Options

While painful and unsightly, most sties heal within a few days on their own or with simple treatment. Chalazions, too, often disappear on their own, but it might take a month or more.

If sties recur, your doctor may prescribe an antibiotic ointment or solution. Apply it to the eyelid (with your eye closed) as directed.

Although a chalazion will often disappear on its own, applying warm compresses to the lid and perhaps a corticosteroid ointment will help speed the process.

In some especially problematic cases that do not respond to home treatment, you may need to have an internal sty or a chalazion removed surgically. An ophthalmologist can perform this minor procedure in the office using a local anesthetic. The eyelid usually heals quickly.

■ Acupuncture
In traditional Chinese medicine it is believed that all types of boils, including sties, are caused by heat invasion.

■ Ayurvedic Medicine
An infusion made with Indian basil can be soaked

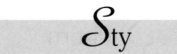

Sty

in a piece of clean cloth or cotton ball and applied to the sty to provide relief. Be sure to read the caution at left about applying treatments to the eye. Consult a qualified practitioner of Ayurvedic medicine for further specific advice.

■ Flower Remedy
Bach Rescue Remedy cream, applied directly to the sty, may help the eyelid heal faster. Be careful when you apply the cream—avoid getting it in your eye.

■ Herbal Therapies
To help reduce the pain and inflammation of sties, herbalists recommend professionally prepared eye drops made from eyebright *(Euphrasia officinalis)*. They may also prescribe an oral preparation of burdock *(Arctium lappa)*.

■ Hydrotherapy
Hydrotherapy treatment for a sty consists of applying hot compresses to the affected eye for 10 to 15 minutes four times daily for several days. This not only relieves pain and inflammation but also helps the sty ripen faster. To make a hot compress, use a cotton cloth or washcloth. Soak it in hot water,

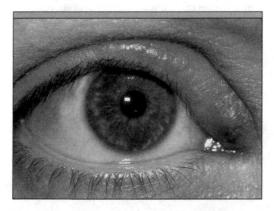

Sty • *A sty results from a bacterial infection at the root of an eyelash, typically at the inner corner of the eye. It causes the follicle of the eyelash to become inflamed (above); a pus-filled bump will form and then rupture. A sty can be painful, but it typically clears up on its own within a week.*

then wring it out; the cloth should be dry enough not to drip but wet enough to maintain a hot temperature for several minutes. Replace or remoisten the cloth as needed to keep it hot. Be sure to close your eye while you apply the compress. When the sty comes to a head, continue applying hot compresses to relieve pressure and promote rupture. Do not squeeze the sty; let it burst on its own.

■ Nutrition and Diet
If you have recurrent sties and chalazions, a nutritionist may recommend that you take supplements of vitamins A and C, which seem to promote healthy skin. You might also want to try a system-cleansing diet, consuming only raw fruits and vegetables, yogurt, herbal teas, fruit juices, and mineral water for up to a week. Naturopathic physicians believe that this diet, repeated at regular intervals, may keep sties from developing.

Home Remedies

The simplest—and often the most effective—treatment for sties and chalazions is to apply hot compresses, as described under Hydrotherapy, above. When the sty has come to a head, it will spontaneously rupture. You can also make a compress by wetting a tea bag with warm water and placing it on your eyelid, with your eye closed, for five minutes three to four times a day.

Prevention

If sties tend to recur, you need to cleanse the outside of your eyelids daily. Put a few drops of very mild baby shampoo into a teacup of warm water and stir. Using a clean cotton swab, gently brush the mixture over your eyelid once a day, keeping your lids closed. It is very important that you avoid contact of the eyelid with cosmetics, dirty towels, or contaminated hands.

Frequent application of hot compresses at the first sign of an infection will prevent further blockage of the lid glands. To keep the infection from spreading to other members of your household, be sure to use a clean, disposable cloth for compresses and do not share washcloths or towels. ■

Sunburn

Symptoms

- Mildly reddish to severely red or purplish skin discoloration; skin feels hot and tender. Sunburn appears one to six hours after exposure to sunlight and peaks within 24 hours, later fading to tan or brown.

- Small, fluid-filled blisters that may itch and eventually break; flaking or peeling skin that reveals the tender, reddened underlayer.

- Red, blistered skin accompanied by chills, fever, nausea, or dehydration. This severe stage of sunburn is considered a first-degree burn.

- Pain and irritation of the eye associated with overexposure to ultraviolet rays from sunlight or other sources.

Call Your Doctor If

- your sunburn blisters and is accompanied by chills, fever, or nausea. Severe sunburn requires professional care in order to limit the risk of infection and to prevent dehydration.

- your eyes are extremely painful and feel gritty. You should have your eyes examined by an ophthalmologist to determine whether the corneas are damaged.

E*ven though light-skinned people have the highest risk of getting sunburned, skin of any color can be damaged by the sun's rays. A sunburn is like any other kind of burn, except that it comes on more slowly. Skin that is reddened and feels hot to the touch can be self-treated and will heal in a matter of days. Sunburned skin that swells or blisters, causing localized pain and overall discomfort, is considered a first-degree burn. A sunburn that results in swelling and extensive blisters may be accompanied by fever, nausea, and dehydration.*

Getting a severe sunburn early in life increases the risk of developing malignant melanoma, a type of skin cancer, years later. (See Rashes and Skin Problems, pages 110-113.)

The Sun's Dangerous Rays

Of the sun's ultraviolet (UV) radiation that penetrates Earth's atmosphere, UVA radiation generally only tans but may also take part in premature aging and wrinkling. UVB rays cause sunburn and the potential for skin cancer. Reflected sunlight from sand, water, or snow is as strong as direct sunlight; shade, clouds, clothes, sunglasses, and sunscreens do not provide complete protection. In addition, certain drugs can intensify the harmful effects of UV radiation; if you are concerned about the potential danger, ask your healthcare practitioner about the risk of photosensitivity.

Treatment Options

Few cases of sunburn require medical care. If the burn is very painful or widespread, a doctor may prescribe oral corticosteroids to relieve the discomfort. Treatment for extremely severe cases of sunburn—those involving extensive blistering, dehydration, or fever—usually requires bed rest and possibly hospitalization.

■ Ayurvedic Medicine
Fresh gel of aloe or a paste made from the herb Indian country mallow can provide relief when they are applied to the skin. A paste or the oil of sandalwood applied to the forehead may help cool the body. Consult a practitioner of Ayurvedic

$\mathcal{S}$unburn

medicine to find out about these and other traditional Indian remedies.

▇ Chinese Medicine

A traditional Chinese remedy for burns of any kind is *Ching Wan Hung* (Beijing Absolute Red); consult a practitioner of Chinese medicine for treatment.

▇ Flower Remedy

The flower remedy known as Rescue Remedy cream can be applied to sunburned skin to provide relief. Consult a practitioner such as a naturopathic physician who is familiar with flower remedies.

▇ Herbal Therapies

Over-the-counter preparations containing aloe *(Aloe barbadensis)* are excellent for relieving the dryness and irritation that accompany sunburn. Lotions, poultices, and compresses containing calendula *(Calendula officinalis)* will reduce inflammation and pain. Echinacea *(Echinacea* spp.) may be used on exposed new skin after peeling or blistering, to help prevent infection.

▇ Homeopathy

Cantharis (12x) taken orally every three to four hours for up to two days is recommended for relieving pain and helping to heal blisters.

▇ Hydrotherapy

A cool bath laced with several tablespoonfuls of baking soda or cider vinegar can relieve the pain, itching, and inflammation of a moderate sunburn.

Home Remedies

Apply cold compresses or calamine lotion to ease itchiness, take aspirin to relieve pain, and have a cool bath or shower for overall relief. Drink plenty of water, but avoid alcohol, which dehydrates the skin. Do not break any blisters; doing so will slow the healing process and increase the risk of infection. When your skin peels or the blisters break, gently remove dried fragments and apply an antiseptic ointment or hydrocortisone cream to the skin beneath. If you feel feverish or nauseated, drink lots of fluids and see a doctor immediately.

Prevention

The most effective way to prevent sunburn is to limit your exposure to direct sunlight, especially between 10:00 a.m. and 3:00 p.m. Take a look at your shadow: If it's shorter than your height, stay under cover.

- If you have to be outside in the midday sun, wear loose-fitting clothes, a broad-brimmed hat, and socks and shoes to protect your feet and ankles.
- Note that radiation exposure is greater at higher altitudes and southern latitudes.
- Any water surface reflects the sun's rays and can double the radiation dose. Protect your skin with a water-resistant sunscreen.
- Protect babies' sensitive skin from strong sunlight, and alert older children to the hazards of overexposure.
- Wear sunglasses that are rated for UV protection. In general, gray, brown, and green lenses—in order from most to least effective—can block out damaging UV rays. ▇

OF SPECIAL INTEREST

Screening the Sun

Two types of sunscreens are on the market. Physical sunblocks, such as zinc ointment, protect by creating a barrier between your skin and the sun. They're good for small areas, such as the nose and lips, but not for your whole body. Products containing para-aminobenzoic acid (PABA) block virtually all UVB rays—the kind most likely to cause sunburn—but offer only minimal protection against UVA rays.

Sunscreens carry a sun protection factor (SPF); a rating of SPF 15 is recommended for most people, but fair-skinned people who are in the sun all day need more. Apply sunscreen 30 minutes before you go out, and reapply it after a swim. Even if you don't swim, a waterproof sunscreen has more staying power. If PABA gives you a rash, try sunscreens containing cinnamates for UVB protection and avobenzone for UVA protection.

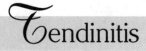

Tendinitis

Symptoms

- Painful tenderness at or near a joint, especially around a shoulder, wrist, or heel (where it is known as Achilles tendinitis), or on the outside of an elbow (where it is called tennis elbow).

- In some cases, numbness or tingling.

- Stiffness that, along with the pain, restricts the movement of the joint involved.

- Occasionally, mild swelling at the joint.

- Persistence of the soreness, which may last or recur long after the tendon has had time to recover from the original injury.

Call Your Doctor If

- your pain doesn't ease up in seven to 10 days. You want to avoid letting chronic tendinitis set in; moreover, you may have another problem such as bursitis, carpal tunnel syndrome, phlebitis, or tenosynovitis.

- your pain is extremely severe and is accompanied by swelling and loss of function. You may have a ruptured tendon, which requires immediate medical attention.

CAUTION

If you have suffered a stroke or have diabetes, circulatory problems, or heart disease, avoid massage and applications of heat or cold until you consult your doctor.

T endinitis is an inflammation in or around a tendon, which is a cable of fibrous tissue that connects a muscle to a bone and transmits the force the muscle exerts. Tendons are designed to withstand bending, stretching, and twisting, but they can become inflamed because of overuse, disease, or injuries that leave them with torn fibers or other damage. The pain can be significant, and it will worsen if the damage progresses because of continued use of the joint. Most tendinitis heals in about two weeks, but chronic tendinitis can take more than six weeks to improve, often because the sufferer doesn't give the tendon time to heal.

Treatment Options

The goal of treatment is to restore movement to the joint without pain and to maintain strength in surrounding muscles while giving the tissues time to heal. Adequate rest is crucial. Returning too soon to the activity that caused the injury can lead to chronic tendinitis or torn tendons.

Ayurvedic Medicine
A paste of Indian bdellium applied directly to the affected area can help soothe the pain of tendinitis.

Body Work
The Alexander technique—which teaches patients how to maintain good body alignment and reduce muscle tension—can have a healing effect on chronic tendinitis. The Feldenkrais method, Rolfing, and Aston-Patterning are other bodywork techniques that may also help heal chronic tendinitis.

Chinese Medicine
Acupuncture, if performed by a qualified practitioner, can be useful in treating tendinitis. A number of Chinese herbal liniments can also soothe tendinitis pain, including *Po Sum On* Medicated Oil, *Tieh Ta Yao Gin* (Traumatic Injury Medicine), and *Zheng Gu Shui*. Chinese herbalists might prepare a poultice of gardenia *(Gardenia jasminoides)*, flour, and wine, which, together with *tui na*—a type of massage that uses the ball of the thumb to manipulate the area—may help to reduce swelling and to increase circulation.

*T*endinitis
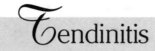

Tendon Injury

Wrist movement is controlled in part by the ex-tensor carpi radialis brevis muscle. If the extended wrist meets a resisting force, as when hitting a ball with a tennis racket, the pressure and stress can cause a muscle tear (inset). Pain and swelling typically follow.

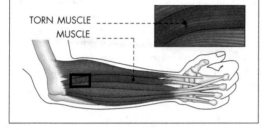

TORN MUSCLE
MUSCLE

■ **Herbal Therapies**

For pain, a naturopathic practitioner might suggest white willow *(Salix alba),* the natural form of as-pirin, taken orally. Try comfrey *(Symphytum offici-nale)* salve, applied two or three times a day, to help relieve inflammation and to strengthen the tendon. Bromelain, an enzyme found in pineapples, is sometimes taken orally with the aim of reducing inflammation in soft tissues; bromelain should not be taken with meals, so take it at least 30 minutes before, or two hours after, eating.

■ **Hydrotherapy**

Use alternating hot and cold compresses: Soak one washcloth in hot water and another in cold. Wring out the warm cloth and place it over the affected area for three minutes; follow with the cold cloth for 30 seconds. Alternate them two more times, fin-ishing with a cold cloth. Do this once or twice a day, as needed.

Or try a hot vinegar pack: Heat equal parts vinegar and water, then soak a towel in the mixture. Wring it out and apply it to the affected area for five minutes. Remove it, then apply a cold one for five minutes. Cover with wool. Repeat these hot-cold applications three times, finishing with cold.

■ **Massage**

If performed by a skilled practitioner, massage can help relieve tendinitis and promote the proper healing of the affected tissues; the friction tech-nique is particularly effective for chronic tendinitis.

■ **Nutrition and Diet**

Research suggests that vitamin supplements may help heal tendinitis. Ask your doctor about taking daily supplements of vitamin C (1,000 mg), beta carotene (vitamin A, 10,000 IU), zinc (22.5 mg), vi-tamin E (400 IU), and selenium (50 mcg).

Home Remedies

Try the RICE treatment: rest, ice, compression, and elevation. Rest mainly means not using the joint, especially not for the same action that injured it. For ice, a bag of frozen vegetables will do if no ice pack is handy. Compression is best provided by an elastic sports bandage wrapping the area snugly, but not painfully tight. For elevation—to reduce flu-id pressure in the injured area—put your ankle on a footstool or lift your elbow onto a chairside table.

Prevention

Include warmups, cooldowns, and stretches in your exercise routine. Vary your exercises, and gradually increase their level of difficulty. ■

OF SPECIAL INTEREST

Tendinitis on the Job

If your tendinitis is caused by tasks you perform at work and you cannot rest your injuries while keeping up with your duties, ask your supervisor for help in modifying your work habits. You may want to request a work-site inspection by an ergonomics specialist, who can analyze the situation and suggest changes. Try some stretches before and after work, and plan to take a five- to 10-minute period each hour to rest the injured area by undertaking tasks that do not involve its use.

Tonsillitis

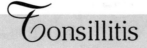

Symptoms

For tonsillitis:

- A very sore throat with red, swollen tonsils; there may be a white discharge or spots on the tonsils.

- Swollen and tender lymph nodes in the neck under the jaw.

- A low-grade fever and headache accompanying the other symptoms.

For tonsillar abscess:

- In addition to inflamed tonsils, severe pain and tenderness around the area of the soft palate, at the roof of the mouth, and difficulty swallowing.

- Distinctively muffled speech, as if the child is speaking with a mouthful of mashed potatoes, caused by swelling from the abscess.

Call Your Doctor If

- your child has symptoms of tonsillitis.

- your child has tonsillitis and starts drooling or having difficulty breathing, which may indicate a tonsillar abscess or epiglottitis, inflammation of the epiglottis. Call 911 or your emergency number now.

- your child has trouble breathing at night or experiences noisy breathing or episodes of sleep apnea, in which the child stops breathing for brief periods while asleep; these symptoms may indicate adenoid problems or overgrown tonsils.

- your child has recurrent bouts of tonsillitis; surgery may be indicated.

T he tonsils are masses of lymphatic tissue located at the back of the throat. They produce antibodies designed to help your child fight respiratory infections. When these tissues themselves become infected, the resulting condition is called tonsillitis. Most tonsil infections and tonsillar abscesses in elementary school age children are caused by the streptococcal bacterium, the same organism that causes strep throat.

Tonsillitis most commonly affects children between the ages of three and seven, when tonsils may play their most active infection-fighting role. But as the child gets older, the tonsils shrink, and infections become less common. Tonsillitis is usually not serious unless a tonsillar abscess develops. When this happens, the swelling can be severe enough to block your child's breathing. Secondary ear infections (otitis media) and adenoid problems are other possible complications.

Treatment Options

Some alternative therapies are effective in relieving the symptoms of tonsillitis. But be sure to first get a throat culture to rule out strep throat, which must be treated with antibiotics. Severe cases may warrant a tonsillectomy. A tonsillar abscess should be treated by a medical doctor before you start any alternative method.

Aromatherapy
A practitioner may recommend oregano and general treatment with a variety of essential oils.

Ayurvedic Medicine
The combined formula *Septilin* may be useful in treating tonsillitis. Other appropriate remedies include an infusion of mint; a powder of the fruit of beleric myrobalan mixed with honey; and a powder or pill of Indian bdellium.

Chinese Medicine
A practitioner of Chinese medicine may advise acupressure to relieve a sore throat, or acupuncture to combat chronic tonsillitis. Often-used herbal remedies include Honeysuckle and Forsythia Powder, thought to help soothe a sore throat in the early stages of tonsillitis; Superior Sore Throat Powder; and *Liu Shen Wan* (Six Spirit Pills).

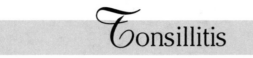

Tonsillitis

Herbal Therapies

To reduce inflammation, herbalists suggest drinking a tea made from cleavers (*Galium* spp.): Add 1 tsp dried herb to 1 cup boiling water. A gargle made from sage *(Salvia officinalis)* is thought to help fight infection: Add 2 tsp to boiling water and steep for 10 minutes. Let your child gargle with the tea (as warm as she can tolerate it) for five minutes several times a day; make sure she does not swallow the tea. The steam from ginger *(Zingiber officinale)* tea may help shrink inflamed tonsils: Breathe in the steam for five minutes, three to four times a day.

Homeopathy

After determining if your child is suffering from acute or chronic tonsillitis, a homeopath may recommend one of the following remedies: for inflamed tonsils, *Belladonna, Hepar sulphuris,* or *Mercurius vivus*; for chronic enlarged tonsils, *Baryta carbonica* or *Calcarea carbonica.*

Hydrotherapy

A hydrotherapist may recommend one or several of the following treatment techniques: tonsillar irrigation; a hot fomentation to the throat, neck, and mastoid; or a heating compress to the throat. Another remedy is known as warming socks: If your child's feet are cold, let her soak them in warm water for five to 10 minutes. Next, soak a pair of cotton socks in cold water and wring them out thoroughly. Place the cold, wet socks on her feet and cover them with dry wool socks. Let her go to bed, being careful to keep her from getting chilled. In the morning, the cotton socks should be dry.

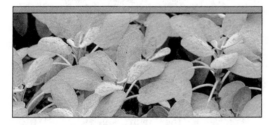

Sage • *The gray-green leaves of sage contain antiseptic and astringent components that may help fight the infection and relieve the discomfort of tonsillitis.*

Osteopathy

Osteopaths treat tonsillitis and tonsillar abscesses with the same surgical and drug therapies offered by conventional medical doctors but may also try gentle soft-tissue manipulation techniques to encourage lymphatic drainage.

Home Remedies

- A salt-water gargle can relieve soreness. Dissolve ½ tsp salt in a glass of warm water and let the child gargle as needed to ease pain. Tell your child not to swallow this solution.
- Ice cream or frozen yogurt after a tonsillectomy will relieve soreness.
- A cool-mist humidifier will increase moisture in the room and soothe a child's sore throat. Aim the mist away from your child so that it does not spray directly at her face, and change her clothes if they become damp. ∎

The Tonsils

Tonsils are lymph nodes at the back of the mouth on either side of the uvula, or soft palate. These small, pinkish lumps of tissue redden and swell when infected, and may develop gray or yellow spots. During an attack of tonsillitis, the glands around the neck under the jaw may feel swollen and tender.

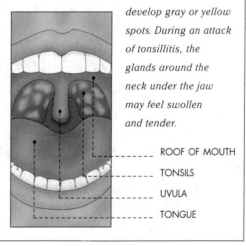

ROOF OF MOUTH

TONSILS

UVULA

TONGUE

Toothache

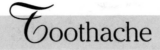

Symptoms

- Aching or sharp pain in tooth when biting or chewing.
- Soreness in teeth, gums, or jaw.

Call Your Dentist If

- your gums are painful, red, and swollen; you may have an impacted tooth or a gum disease. *(See Gum Problems.)*
- you experience continuous bouts of throbbing pain in a tooth, or the tooth is extremely sensitive to heat or cold; you may have tooth decay (a cavity) that requires a new or replacement filling. If the decay is advanced, you may need root canal work. You may also have a tooth abscess, a serious infection requiring emergency treatment.
- you have a sharp pain in your tooth, your tooth feels long or loose, and you have a fever. See your dentist immediately; you may have a tooth abscess.

A toothache can be caused by something as simple as a piece of food wedged between your gum and your tooth—in which case relief involves no more than rinsing or flossing away whatever is causing the pain. But if the pain is not so easily eliminated, you probably have a dental disorder that can cause serious problems if you don't visit your dentist.

The major cause of tooth decay is dental plaque—a substance composed of the bacteria, acids, and sugars in your mouth—which corrodes the protective enamel on your teeth. Initially, you may have no symptoms; but as decay develops, you may feel stabbing pain whenever you eat something hot, cold, sweet, or sour. If decay goes untreated, bacteria infect the underlying dentin and eventually the pulp, or fleshy core, of the tooth. To fight infection, pus floods the pulp, causing a painful tooth abscess. If left untreated, abscesses can damage the jawbone or sinuses and lead to blood poisoning.

Other causes of dental pain include impacted teeth and gum disease (see Gum Problems). Toothaches may also be caused by pressure from sinus congestion, by tooth grinding, or by a blow to the face.

Treatment Options

Alternative remedies may help alleviate the discomfort of symptoms, but conventional treatment is absolutely necessary to stop decay or infection from spreading. You must see a dentist for aches that you suspect may be related to tooth decay; in most cases, the dentist will remove the decayed portion and fill the cavity with a durable material. If the decay is serious, you may need a root canal, which involves removing the pulp, sealing the opening, and then capping the tooth with a crown. If the damage is so severe that a root canal is impossible, or if a tooth is impacted, extraction is the usual treatment. Alternative treatments may ease the pain in the meantime.

Acupressure
Apply deep pressure to the webbing between the index finger and the thumb (Large Intestine 4) to relieve dental pain. Do not press this point if you are pregnant. Massaging this area with an ice cube may also help.

Toothache

Aromatherapy

The essential oils of clove and niaouli *(Melaleuca viridiflora),* applied to the area around the painful tooth, may help soothe a toothache. Be careful to avoid touching oil of clove to the skin, as it may irritate it or cause an allergic reaction.

Ayurvedic Medicine

Applied directly to the affected tooth, the following remedies may bring pain relief: oil from the flowers of cloves; a mixture of ginger, cardamom, and licorice; or paste or oil of sesame seeds.

Chinese Medicine

Acupuncture can often help soothe a toothache. Chinese herbal remedies frequently used for relief from acute dental pain include *Liu Shen Wan* (Six Spirit Pills), *Huang Lien Shang Ching Pien,* and Bezoar Antidotal Tablets.

Flower Remedy

The Bach Rescue Remedy is often recommended for toothache. Consult a naturopath or other practitioner familiar with flower remedies.

Herbal Therapies

Rubbing clove oil *(Syzygium aromaticum)* or myrrh *(Commiphora molmol)* on the gum around a painful tooth can help numb the area.

Homeopathy

Homeopaths often recommend *Hypericum* (12x) and *Arnica* (12x) for relief of toothache. Consult your homeopathic practitioner for other remedies.

Hydrotherapy

Depending on the circumstances of your case, a practitioner may recommend placing an ice pack or hot-water bottle on the jaw near the tooth.

Massage

Gentle massage to the head and face can help relieve pain and tension associated with a toothache.

Home Remedies

Try the following remedies to relieve your pain:
- Rinse with salt water; if this doesn't work, floss gently to pry out any trapped particles.
- Numb your gums: Sucking on ice numbs the gum surrounding a painful tooth.
- Keep cool: Though a hot compress may ease pain, if your toothache is caused by an infection, heat will cause the disease to spread.

Prevention

- Brush and floss after eating; use a nonabrasive, fluoride-based toothpaste. Beware of so-called whitening agents; they often contain abrasives that can wear down enamel.
- Cut down on sweets and carbohydrates. ■

Tooth Decay

Plaque buildup can erode a tooth's protective enamel, causing decay and infection of the underlying dentin. If left untreated, the infection can spread to the pulp, or fleshy core, of the tooth. As the body attempts to fight the infection, a painful, pus-filled abscess may form at the root of the tooth, possibly causing damage to the gum, jawbone, or even the sinuses.

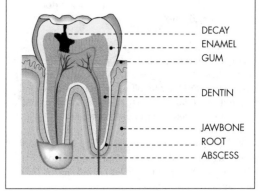

DECAY
ENAMEL
GUM

DENTIN

JAWBONE
ROOT
ABSCESS

Vaginal Problems

Symptoms

- Your vulva is inflamed and it itches; you may have vulvitis.

- The skin of the vulva is thick and has developed white patches; this may indicate a condition called lichen sclerosis or cancer of the vulva. See your doctor for diagnosis.

- Increased vaginal discharge with an offensive odor and burning, itching, and pain; you may have vaginitis.

- You have been sexually or psychologically abused and experience muscle constriction and pain at any attempt to penetrate the vagina; you may have vaginismus.

- An abnormal discharge, bleeding, and/or a firm lesion on any portion of the vagina; you may have vaginal cancer.

Call Your Doctor If

- your bleeding is not caused by menstruation. If you are taking oral contraceptives, it may only be breakthrough bleeding. Otherwise, you may have dysfunctional uterine bleeding. If you are pregnant, there may be a complication in the pregnancy. Postmenopausal bleeding sometimes indicates uterine cancer.

- you have lower abdominal pain along with fever, menstrual disturbances, abnormal discharge, and/or painful sex. You may have a pelvic infection.

- you use tampons, a diaphragm, or a contraceptive sponge and you develop a high fever or rash. You may have toxic shock syndrome.

T *he vagina is the part of the female reproductive system that connects the cervix (the entrance to the uterus) with the vulva, the skin folds that enclose the urethral and vaginal openings. This elastic, muscular passage is lubricated by its own secretions and by mucus-producing glands in the cervix.*

"Vaginitis" is an umbrella term meaning inflammation of the vagina. Yeast causes vaginal yeast infections, the most common form of the disorder. Other vaginal infections include bacterial vaginosis—in which a change in the balance of naturally occurring bacteria in the vagina allows disease-causing bacteria to dominate—and sexually transmitted diseases such as gonorrhea, trichomoniasis, and chlamydia.

The various types of vaginal cancer include squamous cell carcinoma and clear cell adenocarcinoma. Once cancer appears on the vagina, it may spread to surrounding tissues, including the bladder, rectum, vulva, and pubic bone.

Vaginismus is a sexually related psychological disorder. The spasming of the muscles may be painful, interfering with penile penetration or the insertion of other objects such as a speculum or tampon. Sufferers of this disorder usually fear sexual intercourse and associate it with pain.

Treatment Options

Treatment for most vaginal disorders is aimed at maintaining proper bacterial balance and soothing your discomfort. Alternative methods can often help relieve symptoms or ease recovery. But if you have vaginal problems, especially if they are severe or chronic, it is important that you see a doctor for diagnosis and care.

Herbal Therapies

Incorporate fresh garlic *(Allium sativum)* into your diet; it has antibacterial, antifungal, and antiviral properties and may be effective in treating vaginitis, including vaginal yeast infections. You can also try a douche made with goldenseal *(Hydrastis canadensis)* tea.

If itching or minor irritation is a symptom of your vaginitis, bathe with an infusion of fresh chickweed *(Stellaria media)* for relief. (Pour 1 cup of boiling water on 1 to 2 tsp of the herb, steep for

Vaginal Problems

five minutes, and let cool.) To reduce inflammation associated with vulvitis and infectious discharge of bacterial vaginosis, an herbal douche may bring relief. To make, pour 1 cup of boiling water over 1 to 2 tsp of calendula *(Calendula officinalis)* and steep for 10 to 15 minutes; let cool before using the tea as a douche.

Homeopathy

The following remedies taken three or four times a day for one or two days may be used for minor vaginal problems. A smelly, yellow discharge with severe burning, swelling, and soreness may be treated with *Kreosotum* (12c); for itching and a white or yellow discharge, *Sepia* (12c) is recommended; *Pulsatilla* (12c) may aid in treating a thick, creamy yellow-green discharge. See a professional homeopathic practitioner if your condition does not clear up.

Many over-the-counter homeopathic mixtures to treat vaginal yeast infections are available under brand names at your local drugstore.

Lifestyle

If you have recurrent vaginal infections, discontinue the use of tampons for six months. In addition, avoid sexual intercourse while your symptoms of vaginal yeast infection or bacterial vaginosis are still apparent.

OF SPECIAL INTEREST

Products That Can Irritate

Many women may not be aware that their itching and burning may be caused by irritation from products such as soaps, bath oils and crystals, spermicides, swimming pool chlorine, feminine-hygiene sprays, perfumed douches or lubricants, latex products, scented or colored toilet paper, or perfumed pads and tampons. If your physician cannot detect the cause of your irritation, then an allergy or sensitivity to these commercial products is the likely culprit. Stop using suspect items. Try cool soaks in a tub and add Epsom salt if desired.

Wearing cotton panties and avoiding pantyhose and tight clothing will aid in keeping the vagina cool and dry, which may help prevent vulvitis and certain forms of vaginitis.

Nutrition and Diet

If you are susceptible to yeast infections, eating yogurt containing active cultures may help to maintain the natural bacterial flora of the vagina.

Women with recurrent yeast infections should be checked for diabetes. Too much sugar in the diet—whether refined or natural—creates an environment in the vagina that is conducive to the growth of yeast. By removing sugar from your diet, you are in essence starving the yeast.

Home Remedies

Incorporating *Lactobacillus acidophilus* into your diet may be helpful for treating vaginal yeast infections. A paste can be made from refrigerated capsules, available at health food and nutrition stores. Pour the *Lactobacillus acidophilus* powder into your palm and add water to create a pasty substance that may be introduced into the vagina using a vaginal applicator or your finger.

Regular sexual intercourse in postmenopausal women may help prevent dryness and thinning of the vaginal walls, which could increase the likelihood of vaginitis. The activity stimulates blood flow in the area, which keeps vaginal tissue supple.

Prevention

Maintaining good hygiene and using condoms may help prevent vaginitis. If you suspect a vaginal infection, do not douche for 24 hours before seeing your physician, as this may wash away secretions that aid in the diagnosis of your disorder.

A true case of vaginismus is caused by fear rather than by physical abnormality. The best prevention for this disorder is a healthy home environment where sexuality is not made to seem dirty but rather, when appropriate, is discussed in an open, honest, and factual manner. If you have suffered sexual abuse or trauma, you should seek professional help. ■

Varicose Veins

Symptoms

- Prominent dark blue blood vessels, especially in the legs and feet.

- Aching, tender, heavy, or sore legs, often accompanied by swelling in the ankles or feet after standing for any length of time.

- Bulging, ropelike, bluish veins indicate superficial varicose veins.

- Aching and heaviness in a limb, sometimes with swelling, but without any prominent or visible blue vein, may signal a deep varicose vein.

- Discolored, peeling skin; skin ulcers; and constant rather than intermittent pain are signs of severe varicose veins.

Call Your Doctor If

- swelling becomes incapacitating, or the skin over your varicose veins becomes flaky, ulcerous, discolored, or prone to bleeding. You may want to have the veins removed to avoid potentially worse problems.

- you have red varicose veins. This may be a sign of phlebitis, a serious circulatory condition.

- you have continuing pain with no outward signs. Contact a doctor at once about the possibility of deep varicose veins.

- you cut a varicose vein. Control the resulting burst of blood and have the vein treated to prevent complications.

V aricose veins usually announce themselves as bulging, bluish cords running just beneath the surface of your skin. They can appear anywhere in the body but most often affect legs and feet, particularly in women. Visible swollen and twisted veins—sometimes surrounded by patches of flooded capillaries known as spider-burst veins—are considered superficial varicose veins. Although they can be painful and disfiguring, they are usually harmless. On rare occasions, an interior leg vein becomes varicose. Deep varicose veins are usually not visible, but they can cause swelling or aching throughout the leg.

Treatment Options

Aromatherapy

Oils of cypress and German chamomile (Matricaria recutita) may soothe swelling and inflammation and help relieve pain.

Chiropractic

To treat varicose veins, chiropractic medicine combines diet and lifestyle therapy with physical manipulation of the skeletal system. Manipulation to relieve strain on the pelvis, for example, is intended to improve the flow of blood and other fluids through the body.

Exercise

Aerobic exercise totaling 30 minutes a day several times a week will help you keep your weight down while toning and strengthening veins. You might start your morning with a brisk walk, for example, or finish your day with a swim or bike ride.

Herbal Therapies

Ginkgo (Ginkgo biloba), hawthorn (Crataegus laevigata), and bilberry (Vaccinium myrtillus) are all reported to strengthen blood vessels and improve peripheral circulation. Tinctures or topical ointments of horse chestnut (Aesculus hippocastanum) and butcher's-broom (Ruscus aculeatus) are also recommended for toning veins while reducing inflammation; butcher's-broom can also be prepared as tea. For skin irritation associated with varicose veins, try a lotion made of distilled witch hazel (Hamamelis virginiana).

Varicose Veins

■ Homeopathy

For immediate relief from specific symptoms, you can try over-the-counter homeopathic remedies: *Hamamelis,* or witch hazel, cream in a 6x to 15c solution applied to an area that is bluish and perhaps bruised may relieve soreness. *Hamamelis* 6x to 15c can also be taken internally as directed on the label for general relief. *Belladonna,* 12x or 12c potency four times a day, is recommended for red, hot, swollen, and tender varicose veins.

■ Hydrotherapy

Sponge or spray legs with cold water to relieve aches and pain from superficial varicose veins. Hot and cold baths may slow the progression of varicose veins on the feet and ankles: Dip your feet in warm water for one to two minutes, then cold water for half a minute, alternating this procedure for 15 minutes.

■ Massage

Regular massage can markedly alleviate discomfort associated with varicose veins. A massage therapist starts at the feet and massages your legs up to the hips and along the lymphatic system to mobilize congested body tissues. Use light pressure when massaging deep or severe varicose veins.

■ Nutrition and Diet

Extra body fat increases water retention and puts pressure on the legs and abdomen, aggravating varicosity. To decrease body fat, eat foods that are low in fat, sugar, and salt, and high in fiber. To promote a healthy flow of nutrients and waste through the body, make fruits, vegetables, and whole grains the mainstays of your diet, and drink plenty of fluids, especially spring water.

Home Remedies

To ease painful swelling and inflammation associated with varicose veins in your legs, rest frequently, wear support stockings, and take one or two aspirin or ibuprofen tablets daily until the condition clears. Cross your legs at the ankles rather than the knees for better circulation. Better yet, take a break and put your feet up; periods of rest with your feet a few inches above your heart level help pooled blood drain from your legs. To further improve circulation, women should wear loose clothing and avoid high heels in favor of flat shoes.

Prevention

- If your daily routine requires you to be on your feet constantly, stretch and exercise your legs as often as possible to increase circulation and reduce pressure buildup.
- If you smoke, quit. Studies show that smoking may contribute to elevated blood pressure, which in turn can aggravate varicosity.
- If you're pregnant, be sure to sleep on your left or right side rather than on your back to minimize pressure from the uterus on the veins in your pelvic area. This position will also improve blood flow to the fetus. ■

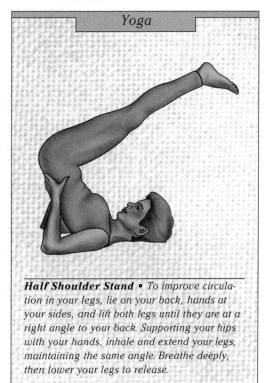

Yoga

Half Shoulder Stand • *To improve circulation in your legs, lie on your back, hands at your sides, and lift both legs until they are at a right angle to your back. Supporting your hips with your hands, inhale and extend your legs, maintaining the same angle. Breathe deeply, then lower your legs to release.*

Warts

Symptoms

- Common warts are small, hard, rough lumps that are round and elevated; they usually appear on hands and fingers and may be flesh colored, white, or pink, and either smooth or granulated.

- Digitate warts are horny and fingerlike, with pea-shaped bases; they appear on the scalp or near the hairline.

- Filiform warts are thin and threadlike; they commonly appear on the face and neck.

- Flat warts appear in groups of up to several hundred, usually on the face, neck, chest, knees, hands, wrists, or forearms; they are slightly raised and have smooth, flat or rounded tops.

- Genital warts are painless flesh-colored or grayish white growths on the vulva, anus, or penis that may develop a cauliflower-like appearance.

- Periungual warts are rough, irregular, and elevated; they appear at the edges of fingernails and toenails and may extend under the nails, causing pain.

- Plantar warts are small, bumpy growths on the soles of the feet, one-quarter inch to two inches in diameter, sometimes with tiny black dots on the surface.

Call Your Doctor If

- over-the-counter remedies or alternative therapies don't work.

- you are a woman and develop genital warts, which in rare cases may indicate cervical cancer.

- you are older than 45 and discover what looks like a wart; it may instead be a symptom of a more serious skin condition, such as skin cancer.

- you notice a change in a wart's color or size; this could indicate skin cancer.

Warts are among the most common dermatological complaints. A certain percentage of them may be caused by the human papilloma virus (HPV), which enters the skin through a cut or scratch and causes cells to multiply rapidly. Usually, warts spread through direct contact, but it is possible to pick up the virus in moist environments, such as showers and locker rooms. You can spread them to other parts of your body by touching them or shaving around infected areas. Children and young adults are more prone to getting warts because their defense mechanisms may not be fully developed, but it is possible to get a wart at any age.

Treatment Options

The best treatment for warts is often no treatment at all; most people develop an immune response that causes warts to go away by themselves. However, if your wart doesn't disappear, or if it's unsightly or uncomfortable, you can try the alternative treatments or home remedies listed here. Over-the-counter medications work by softening abnormal skin cells and dissolving them; your doctor can also remove warts surgically or by freezing or burning them off. Seek your doctor's care for genital warts.

Chinese Medicine

A doctor of Chinese medicine may place a slice of ginger (Zingiber officinale) root on top of the wart and cover it with smoldering mugwort leaf (Artemisia argyi). The burning herb enables the ginger to release its antiviral constituents. This process is called indirect moxibustion.

Herbal Therapies

Several herbs contain chemicals thought to fight viruses and help treat skin conditions. Herbalists recommend applying the sticky juices of dandelion (Taraxacum officinale), milkweed (Asclepias syriaca), and celandine (Chelidonium majus). An ointment of thuja (Thuja occidentalis) applied four or five times a day may also help.

Whichever herbal remedy you try, first protect the surrounding skin with petroleum jelly and then cover the treated wart with a clean bandage. Repeat daily until the wart is gone.

*W*arts

■ Homeopathy
Homeopathic medicines for warts include *Causticum, Nitric acid,* and *Antimonium crudum.*

■ Mind/Body Medicine
Using guided imagery to relax may help speed the immune system's response to warts. Breathe deeply as you imagine the wart dissolving. Do this for five minutes, twice a day; some warts will disappear after one to two months.

■ Nutrition and Diet
Poor diet can be a factor in persistent or recurring warts. Foods high in vitamin A—eggs, cold-water fish, onions, garlic, and dark green and yellow vegetables—will help sustain your immune system, as will yogurt and other fermented-milk products. You can also consult a nutritional therapist about the potential benefits of supplemental vitamins A, B complex, C, and E; L-cysteine; and zinc.

Home Remedies

There are countless folk cures for warts. One that may have some validity is rubbing the wart with a slice of raw potato or the inner side of a banana skin; both contain chemicals that may dissolve the wart. You might also try any of the following applications:

- Vitamins A and E, which are generally good for skin conditions.
- A paste of crushed vitamin C tablets and water.
- Over-the-counter medicines or a paste of crushed aspirin; both contain wart-dissolving salicylic acid.
- Aloe *(Aloe barbadensis),* dandelion, or milkweed juices.
- Cotton soaked in fresh pineapple juice, which contains a dissolving enzyme.

Prevention

Practice good hygiene, and eat balanced meals high in vitamins A, C, and E to boost your immune system. Avoid stress, which can compromise your immunity, and learn to relax. ■

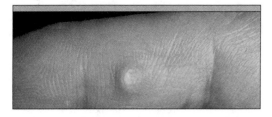

Common Wart • *Typically found on the hands and feet either singly or in clusters, common warts vary in size but average a quarter inch in diameter. The flesh-colored bumps tend to be circular and feel hard and rough to the touch. They pose no health risks and will eventually disappear, but they can also be removed with over-the-counter medications.*

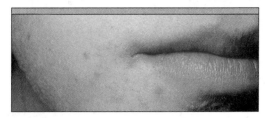

Flat Warts • *Children and young adults are those most likely to develop flat warts, which often occur in clusters of 10 to 30. The warts are slightly raised, smooth, and tan or flesh colored; they are often barely visible. Flat warts typically appear on the neck, face, wrists, backs of the hands, and knees. In children, they most often appear on the face.*

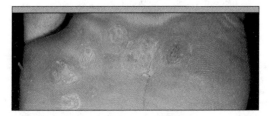

Plantar Warts • *Caused by the common wart virus, plantar warts appear on the sole of the foot, usually at pressure points such as the heel. They begin as small, painful warts that then become flattened and pressed into the skin. The soft core of the wart is surrounded by a hard, calluslike ring that may be peppered with tiny blood clots that appear as black dots.*

*Y*east Infections

Symptoms

- In women, vaginal itching and irritation; redness and swelling of the vulva; unusually thick, white discharge; and pain during intercourse. These are signs of a vaginal yeast infection, also known as moniliasis.

- In men, red patches and blisters at the end of the penis and around the foreskin, possibly with severe itching and pain. These are symptoms of balanitis.

- Painless white patches in your mouth or throat that may come off when you eat or brush your teeth; this indicates oral thrush, which is most common in infants, the elderly, and AIDS patients.

- White patches in the mouth and throat, sometimes associated with painful swallowing; these are symptomatic of esophageal thrush, a potential complication of AIDS.

- Peeling skin on the hands, especially between the fingers; and swollen nail folds above the cuticle, possibly painful, red, and containing pus.

- Itchy or burning shiny pink rash with a scaly or blistered edge in the folds of the skin. This indicates intertrigo.

Call Your Doctor If

- you have any of the symptoms for the first time; you will need a professional evaluation before beginning treatment.

- the infection does not respond to treatment or recurs; you may have a more serious disorder such as diabetes or an HIV infection.

Y *east, or fungal, infection—sometimes called candidiasis—takes many forms. Yeast infections often develop where a moist environment encourages fungal growth, especially on the webs of fingers and toes, nails, genitals, and folds of skin. Oral thrush is a painless, often recurrent infection of the mouth and throat; it is common in babies, young children, and the elderly, but can affect all ages. Moniliasis is a painful vaginal yeast infection experienced by many women, most commonly during pregnancy or treatment with antibiotics. (See Vaginal Problems, pages 134-135.) Balanitis is a less common but equally irritating infection of the penis. Systemic yeast infections can occur in cases of diabetes, AIDS, and other ailments or drug treatments that suppress the immune system.*

What Makes You Susceptible

Candida albicans is a fungal organism, or yeast, that thrives in your mouth, gastrointestinal tract, and skin; your body produces bacterial flora that keeps it in check. When fungal growth exceeds the body's ability to control it, yeast infection develops. This can happen when you are weakened by illness or upset by stress. Modern antibiotics that treat many ailments can actually kill the bacteria that otherwise control fungal outbreaks.

Yeast infections are common among dishwashers and people whose hands are often in water, in children who suck their thumbs or fingers, and in people whose clothing retains body moisture. Diabetics are especially prone to yeast infections because they have high levels of sugar in their blood and urine and a low resistance to infection—conditions that encourage yeast growth.

Treatment Options

Treatment depends on the specific kind of infection you have but should focus on counteracting the growth of the yeast organism. For vaginal yeast infections, an over-the-counter intravaginal cream containing miconazole or clotrimazole usually works well; an oral form is now also available. If over-the-counter medications are not effective, you may need to see a physician, who can prescribe a stronger medication.

Yeast Infections

Chronic Yeast Infection

Although the diagnosis is not universally accepted, some doctors recognize a condition called chronic candidiasis, or chronic yeast infection, that may affect the gastrointestinal, nervous, endocrine, and immune systems. Treatment focuses on eliminating predisposing factors, such as prescription or over-the-counter drugs, foods with high refined-sugar or yeast content, high-carbohydrate vegetables, and milk products. Your doctor may also test you for underlying conditions, such as diabetes or thyroid problems.

*An herbal remedy for chronic yeast infection is tea brewed from 2 to 3 tsp dried root of barberry (Berberis vulgaris) or **goldenseal** (Hydrastis canadensis) in a cup of boiling water, taken three times a day. With your doctor's approval, you may want to try taking daily supplements of 45 mg **iron**, 45 mg **zinc**, and 200 mcg **selenium** (avoid higher doses of selenium).*

Alternative remedies may also be effective. Some are targeted at strengthening the immune system so that your body will be better able to resist yeast infections; others provide symptom relief or aim to treat specific yeast infections and prevent them from recurring.

Ayurvedic Medicine

For vaginal yeast infections, tablets of the combination formula *Septilin* are sometimes given. Another Ayurvedic remedy is a vaginal douche made from an infusion of mugwort. Consult a qualified practitioner of Ayurvedic medicine to get specific information on these and other forms of Ayurvedic treatment.

Chinese Medicine

There are a variety of acupuncture and Chinese herbal treatments for yeast infections. Consult a practitioner of Chinese medicine for a specific diagnosis and treatment regimen.

Herbal Therapies

For healing yeast infections on your skin, apply full-strength tea tree (*Melaleuca* spp.) oil two to three times daily; a slight burning sensation is normal, but discontinue if the treatment is painful. An over-the-counter salve containing calendula (*Calendula officinalis*) is good for rashes in children over two years of age.

For infections caused by a fungus, try pau d'arco (*Tabebuia impetiginosa*). In tincture form, take 15 drops two times a day for a month or two; as a tea, drink 2 cups a day for two to three months. Garlic (*Allium sativum*) can also help fight yeast infections; try two capsules or pills two times a day for two or three months. These remedies may be helpful for chronic infection.

Homeopathy

Numerous homeopathic remedies are used to treat yeast infections; a licensed homeopathic physician will diagnose your condition and can then recommend the best remedies and course of treatment to match your symptoms.

Hydrotherapy

Alternating hot and cold sitz baths may provide symptom relief and help speed recovery from a vaginal yeast infection. To prepare a sitz bath, place a towel in the bottom of a washtub or bathtub, and fill the tub so that the water comes up to about ½ inch above your navel. For these baths, fill one tub with hot water and another with cold; sit in the hot water for about three minutes, then the cold water for about 30 seconds. Do this three times, making sure to end with the cold and dry yourself thoroughly after the treatment.

Prevention

- If work keeps your hands in water for long periods, wear rubber gloves. When you're done, wash your hands and apply a mild prescription or over-the-counter antifungal cream.
- Wear cotton or silk underclothes, which, unlike nylon and other synthetics, allow excess moisture to evaporate. Wash and dry your underclothes thoroughly; change them often. ■

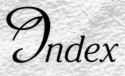

Index

Page numbers in italic refer to illustrations or to illustrated text.